30-MINUTE SIBO COOKBOOK

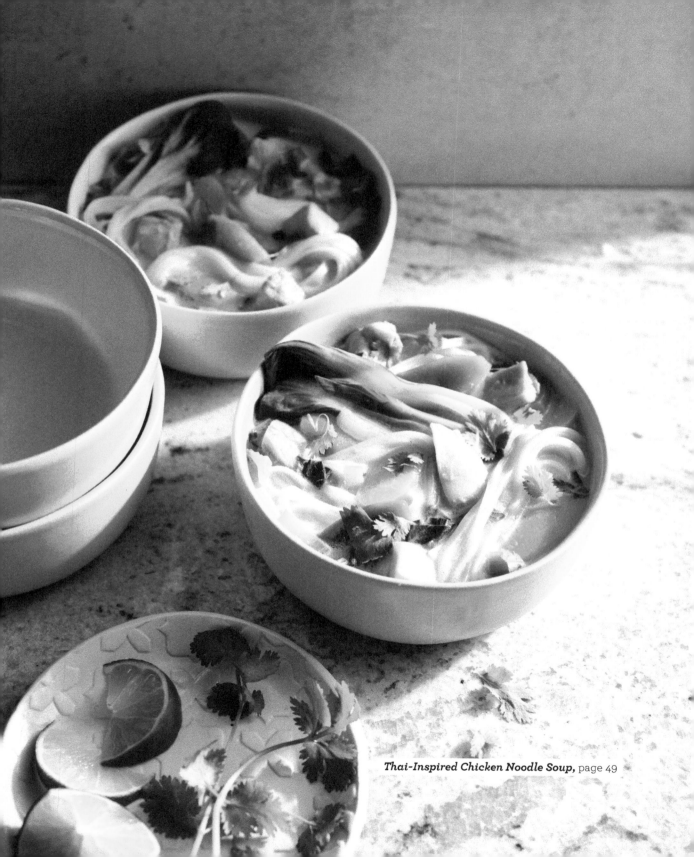

Thai-Inspired Chicken Noodle Soup, page 49

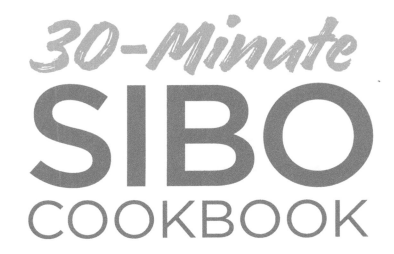

30-Minute SIBO COOKBOOK

65 *Fast Recipes* to Relieve Symptoms

Kristy Regan, MScN

Photography by Iain Bagwell

ROCKRIDGE
PRESS

For general information on our other products and services or to obtain technical support, please contact our Customer Care Department within the United States at (866) 744-2665, or outside the United States at (510) 253-0500.

Rockridge Press publishes its books in a variety of electronic and print formats. Some content that appears in print may not be available in electronic books, and vice versa.

TRADEMARKS: Rockridge Press and the Rockridge Press logo are trademarks or registered trademarks of Callisto Media Inc. and/or its affiliates, in the United States and other countries, and may not be used without written permission. All other trademarks are the property of their respective owners. Rockridge Press is not associated with any product or vendor mentioned in this book.

Interior and Cover Art Director: Antonio Valverde
Art Producer: Karen Williams
Editors: Morgan Shanahan and Claire Yee
Production Editor: Matthew Burnett

Photography © 2020 Iain Bagwell. Food styling by Katelyn Hardwick. Author photo courtesy of © Emily V. Whellbarger.
Cover: Citrus, Shrimp & Rice Salad; page 43

ISBN: Print 978-1-64739-736-4 | eBook 978-1-64739-438-7
R0

*To my family and friends, thank you for being there
through thick and thin.
To Gregg, thank you for being my person.*

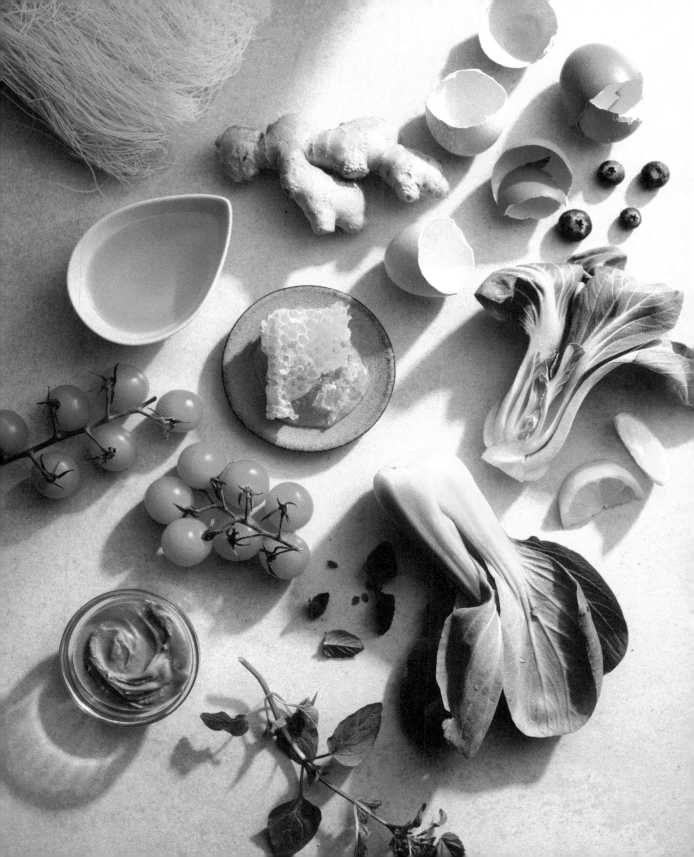

Contents

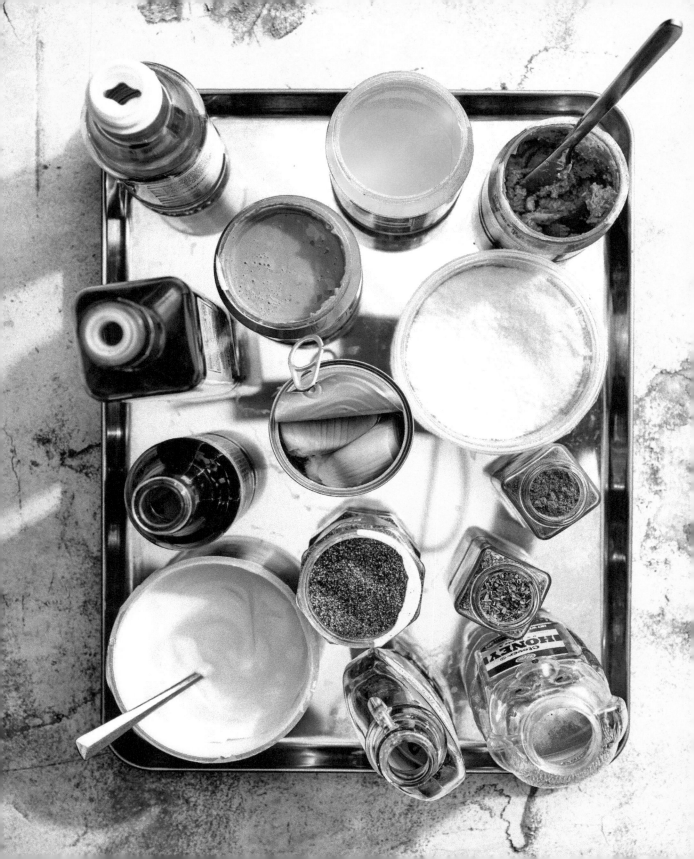

Foreword

I am a naturopathic gastroenterologist, and over the past two decades I have lectured about digestive health and disease. I supervise student doctors who work with patients suffering from complex digestive conditions. I met Kristy about a decade ago, when she was a student in the Master of Science in Nutrition program at the National University of Natural Medicine. She chose to attend weekly one of my clinic rotations, for a year, in order to help our patients with their diets. She was especially focused on diets for SIBO and related conditions. Since her graduation, I have called on her to help many of my patients with the ins and outs of diet, nutrition, cooking, and support. She continues to attend our weekly case conferences and is a great asset to physicians working in the field of functional gastroenterology.

Kristy's first cookbook, *The SIBO Diet Plan*, is a great guide for my patients with bacterial overgrowth and many other digestive issues. Her next book, *The SIBO Cookbook for the Newly Diagnosed*, gives us more recipes to enjoy and additional resources to navigate the essential process of individualizing a diet for those newly diagnosed with SIBO. Now, her *30-Minute SIBO Cookbook* brings us additional, user-friendly, and quickly prepared recipes. Having great recipes that are quick to prepare is important when my patients are making most of their meals from scratch. I appreciate that these cookbooks include diet-specific labels and nutritional labels at the top of each recipe. These labels list the various diets (LFD, SCD, SSFG, etc.) for which the recipe is also appropriate as well as which essential allergenic categories (gluten-free, dairy-free, vegetarian, etc.) it falls under.

I work with many patients dealing with SIBO. Kristy helps them create a personalized, joyous, and tasty diet—despite the restrictions of their digestive conditions. When Kristy writes, "Reset your gut, but enjoy your life," it's the hope for which my patients are searching. In the past few years, many nutritionists have jumped on the SIBO train and have declared themselves "experts" in diet for SIBO. Kristy is the real deal.

Steven Sandberg-Lewis, ND, DHANP
Naturopathic physician
Portland, Oregon, May 2020

Introduction

When I was diagnosed with SIBO in 2012, there weren't any SIBO cookbooks, and it would be a year before Dr. Allison Siebecker published her SIBO Specific Food Guide, the first diet specifically aimed at mitigating SIBO symptoms. My doctor advised me to follow the specific carbohydrate diet (SCD), which showed efficacy for ulcerative colitis and Crohn's disease but hadn't been studied for IBS or SIBO. I fanatically followed that diet for a year and a half but didn't feel better. When I eventually took another SIBO test, I found that my overgrowth had tripled in size.

Over time, I found a diet that worked for me, which was low-FODMAP. FODMAP stands for fermentable oligosaccharides, disaccharides, monosaccharides, and polyols. These are types of fermentable carbohydrates that many people with IBS and SIBO don't tolerate. As part of my health journey, I also established a medical team of SIBO experts who supported me in healing.

Thankfully, we've learned so much about SIBO in the past eight years from a medical perspective, and today there are many more resources for those with SIBO. I'm excited to contribute to the available resources by writing this book. I understand that cooking when you have SIBO can be confusing and frustrating at a time when you're already tired and overwhelmed! This 30-minute-or-less recipe approach will support you in saving time in the kitchen so you can get quick, tasty meals on the table and redirect your energy onto your health.

In this book, I'll introduce a variety of often-tolerated foods that can support you in healing and focus on widely available nutrient-dense fruits, vegetables, proteins, and herbs that add lots of fresh taste.

One mistake people often make in eating for SIBO is to restrict too many foods. Sometimes they end up only eating a couple of foods and then start reacting to those foods. By emphasizing a wider variety of fruit and vegetable consumption, you'll support a healthier microbiome and make eating more enjoyable. I recommend making healthy fats, carbohydrates, and protein a part of every meal. Some recipes will incorporate all three of these macronutrients. For others, I'll make it easy for you to add a side of protein or vegetables. Many people don't always think about adding fat to their meals, but for those with SIBO, it's important to incorporate fats into your diet to keep you satiated and to support the absorption of the fat-soluble vitamins A, D, E, and K.

Of course, there's also an emotional component to being on a therapeutic diet. Many people feel deprived by not eating their favorite foods and even feel like their social life has changed because of food restrictions. If you can relate to this, it can be useful to talk with a nutritionist or other medical provider. A practitioner can help you see patterns in how your diet and symptoms may be related. As you shift to a new way of eating, it's important to find new favorite recipes that you can share with family and friends, and that's where this book comes in. I truly expect that some of these recipes will become ones that you'll want to make again and again.

And here's some more good news: After adopting a SIBO diet, many people experience a large decrease in symptoms. This is life-changing for many people who are severely symptomatic. While it's important to not expect complete elimination of all symptoms without successfully address-ing the underlying cause, you can bring symptoms to a manageable level—all while eating the widest variety of food possible.

This cookbook gives you that variety, along with the ease of cooking a meal in 30 minutes or less. And don't we all need more time and ease in our lives? As you progress, you'll want to add in a greater variety of food, including high-FODMAP foods that don't cause symptoms. Not all people will react to all FODMAPs, so you can add in those that don't cause a reaction.

I hope that through this cookbook, you'll find more joy in the process of both eating and cooking, giving you time for yourself and your relation-ships, along with a well-deserved opportunity to heal and feel good again.

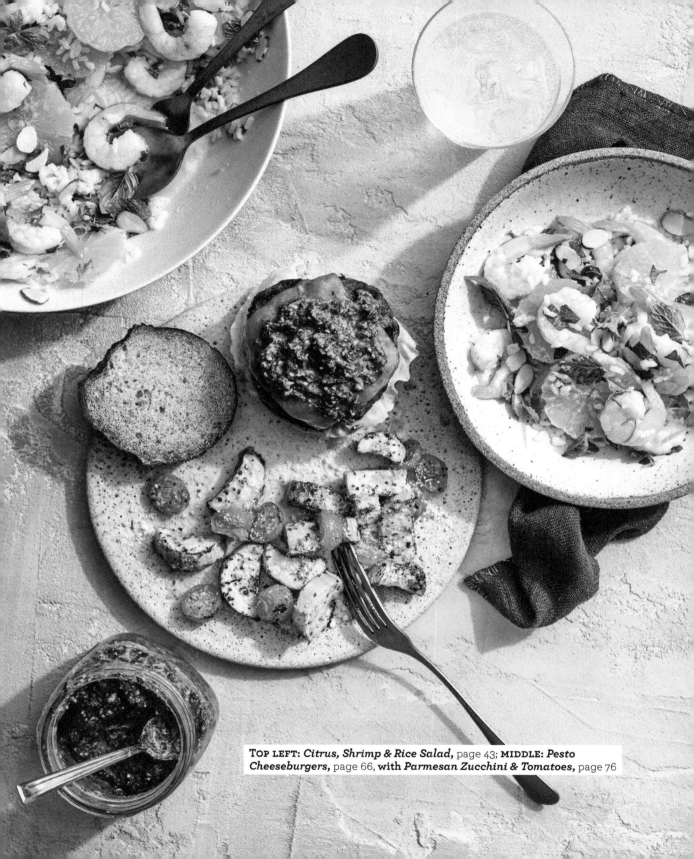

TOP LEFT: *Citrus, Shrimp & Rice Salad,* page 43; MIDDLE: *Pesto Cheeseburgers,* page 66, with *Parmesan Zucchini & Tomatoes,* page 76

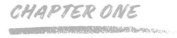
The SIBO-Diet Connection

Having SIBO can be challenging, but this cookbook is here to easily break it down for you. This chapter provides a foundational understanding of SIBO, the different types and symptoms, and how your digestive system is affected by SIBO. We'll explore how to mitigate the symptoms of SIBO with different diets, and you'll learn how to optimize your kitchen to start a SIBO diet and cook from a new, exciting vantage point—that of improving your health! This chapter will set the groundwork for preparing and enjoying all the quick, delicious, and accessible meals offered in this book.

What Is SIBO?

Small intestinal bacterial overgrowth (SIBO) is caused by a bacterial over-growth in the small intestine. The small intestine isn't set up to handle large amounts of bacteria, so an overgrowth can lead to symptoms that may include:

▸ Diarrhea

▸ Constipation

▸ Bloating

▸ Gas and belching

▸ Cramping

▸ Nausea

▸ Food sensitivities

▸ Skin symptoms

▸ Malabsorption

▸ Fatigue

▸ Anxiety

▸ Joint pain

▸ and others

Though some SIBO symptoms are typical for many people, overall symptoms vary for each individual.

The most common way to diagnose SIBO is through a lactulose breath test, which measures hydrogen and methane gases in your breath. Normally, these gases aren't present, but with an overgrowth, they are present and can be measured.

When you're diagnosed with SIBO, it's important to understand why you have it and what the size of the bacterial overgrowth is. Depending on the underlying cause and the size of the bacterial overgrowth, your doctor will present different treatment options. For many people, the underlying cause is food poisoning. Food poisoning creates antibodies that damage the migrating motor complex (see page 5), setting the stage for a bacterial overgrowth. For others, it might be from abdominal surgery and resulting adhesions. And for many people, it's not just SIBO but other concurrent issues, such as candida or small intestine fungal overgrowth (SIFO).

If you have a small overgrowth, the treatment may look different from that for someone who has very high numbers. Some people may have a very mild case of SIBO and eradicate it rather quickly. For others, the journey may be longer and more extensive. Luckily, a SIBO diet can help mitigate symptoms. Lifestyle changes, like addressing stress, may also provide benefits. My clients have told me that even though they never wanted to have SIBO, it has helped them understand their bodily cues better, focus on a healthy long-term diet, and avoid overextending themselves in their everyday lives.

Getting to the point of receiving a SIBO diagnosis can be a frustrating process. Perhaps your doctor hasn't heard of or doesn't believe in SIBO. Thankfully, this is becoming less common as more medical professionals learn about SIBO, but you might need to inform your doctor about SIBO and why you think you have it. Speak to your doctor if you have any of the following key indicators of SIBO, which were introduced by Dr. Steven Sandberg-Lewis and Dr. Allison Siebecker:

▶ You have gas, bloating, diarrhea, or constipation.

▶ Your symptoms worsened after an incident of stomach flu or food poisoning, abdominal surgery, or antibiotic, opiate, or proton pump inhibitor (PPI) use.

▶ You react to foods you used to be able to eat without issue.

▶ You've experienced undesired weight loss even though you're eating the same amount or more.

▶ High fiber or high-FODMAP foods contribute to symptoms.

▶ Taking antibiotics for other reasons decreased your symptoms for a period of time.

▶ You've had to severely restrict your food intake and your variety of foods to control your symptoms.

▶ You have deficiencies such as low vitamin B_{12} or D, anemia, or chronic low ferritin with no other discernible cause.

▶ You take laxatives regularly in order to have a bowel movement.

▶ You've experienced increased anxiety with no other discernible cause in addition to gastrointestinal symptoms.

There are four types of SIBO. Each has its own distinctive challenges and may be treated slightly differently:

Hydrogen dominant SIBO. People with hydrogen dominant SIBO are more likely to have diarrhea and may experience weight loss.

Methane dominant SIBO. People with methane dominant SIBO are more likely to experience constipation and may experience weight gain.

Mixed SIBO. Having mixed SIBO means that both hydrogen and methane gases were detected on your SIBO test. Your symptoms may vary and may include alternating diarrhea and constipation.

Hydrogen sulfide SIBO. Hydrogen sulfide SIBO is currently detected from a flat line (low numbers) SIBO test, with symptoms possibly including foul-smelling gas and diarrhea.

A Quick Breakdown of Your Digestive System

For some, digestion is something that we take for granted until it becomes an issue. For others, digestion has always presented problems and has worsened over time. It's important to understand the basics of digestion and how digestion relates to SIBO in order to understand symptoms. This knowledge will serve as a tool when discussing your health with your doctor and addressing symptoms.

Esophagus

The esophagus typically takes over digestion once you swallow your food. A series of automatic muscle contractions, called peristalsis, takes place in the esophagus, stomach, and intestines to move food through the system. When SIBO is present, people may experience heartburn or acid reflux. Gas from a bacterial overgrowth can cause the esophageal sphincter to open improperly, and stomach acid can flow back into the esophagus, irritating the esophageal lining.

Stomach

The stomach contains gastric acids that inhibit the growth of bacteria in the stomach from bacteria we ingest. Diminished acid production may cause symptoms of nausea, stomach pain, bloating, or a feeling of uncomfortable fullness after meals. Sometimes diminished acid production can be due to aging or use of a proton pump inhibitor (PPI) for acid reflux.

The stomach and small intestine also have a migrating motor complex (MMC), which is a sweeper or housecleaning wave that occurs in both areas during periods of fasting. When the function of the MMC is disturbed due to a variety of issues including food poisoning, an overgrowth can occur in the small intestine.

Gallbladder

The gallbladder, situated in the upper right side of the abdomen, stores bile, which is delivered to the small intestine to break down fat and enables nutrients and fat-soluble vitamins to be easily absorbed. In the case of a bacterial overgrowth, bile can be broken apart, leading to issues with fat breakdown, which in turn can cause fat-soluble vitamin deficiencies and steatorrhea, which is the presence of fat in feces that may be linked to malabsorption. Fat malabsorption can lead to symptoms of nausea or diarrhea after eating fatty foods. Vitamin deficiencies can lead to issues including fatigue, depression, hair loss, brittle nails, and mouth ulcers.

Small Intestine

The small intestine absorbs nutrients and minerals from the food we eat. The small intestine typically houses a smaller number of bacteria than the large intestine. These bacteria protect us against yeast and harmful bacteria. The MMC that's also in the stomach rids the area of undigested debris, which is then moved to the large intestine for excretion.

When the MMC isn't working properly, a bacterial overgrowth can take place. The overgrowth of bacteria consumes nutrients in the small intestine that would typically be absorbed. Gas is then expelled from the bacteria, causing symptoms of bloating, diarrhea, constipation, belching, or flatulence. When the small intestine's lining is damaged from bacteria, food particles may enter the bloodstream, causing food sensitivities.

Large Intestine

The large intestine absorbs water and electrolytes, forms feces, and eliminates them via the rectum. The large intestine is connected to the small intestine via the ileocecal valve. If the ileocecal valve isn't functioning correctly, bacteria from the large intestine can move backward into the small intestine and contribute to an overgrowth. When a bacterial overgrowth is present in the small intestine, normal bowel movements can be disturbed. Diarrhea and constipation are two very common symptoms of SIBO.

THE LOWDOWN ON FEELING LOW

Having a chronic illness that can't be seen and that many people, including doctors, haven't even heard of can take an emotional toll. Many who have SIBO rely on multiple health practitioners, cook most or all of their food, research SIBO and educate themselves and others, track multiple symptoms, and find themselves reevaluating their schedules, social outings, and even careers.

It's not surprising that all of this can increase anxiety, irritability, and fatigue. Symptoms like depression can also be brought on by deficiencies in vitamin D or vitamin B_{12}, both of which can be related to SIBO. Many people with SIBO also experience brain fog, concentration issues, or forgetfulness. However, this is different from an ongoing mental health disorder that should be diagnosed and treated by a professional.

Cooking delicious food and eating well will support your mental health, but being on a SIBO diet may not relieve mental health symptoms. Bring up any mental health issues or symptoms with your doctor, and they will refer you to a mental health specialist as needed. An anxiety disorder can be both diagnosed and treated, and it is different from the general anxiety that is linked to the physical issue of SIBO.

Healing Your Gut in 30 Minutes a Meal

Many people find living with daily symptoms of SIBO challenging, even debilitating. That's why most people use a diet to relieve symptoms. In this cookbook, we follow the low-FODMAP diet. The diet contains a variety of low-FODMAP grains that help those who tolerate them feel less restricted and prevent unintended weight loss. The easy-to-cook recipes in this book are especially delicious and contain a variety of foods. A SIBO diet shouldn't feel punitive, and the goal of this cookbook is to give you quick and tasty food options and, with those, more time to enjoy the other parts of your life. That's why every single recipe in this cookbook can be made in 30 minutes or less. That's a promise!

By adopting a SIBO diet and following some key principles, symptom management is attainable. Here are a few guidelines to help keep you on track:

Start simply and keep a food diary. Choose recipes with few ingredients to determine if you are reacting to particular items. Even if a food is on the approved diet, you may still react to it. For instance, some people can consume starchy foods such as white rice or white potato, while others don't tolerate such foods. This is unique to the individual, so keeping a food diary in the beginning will help you make connections between foods and symptoms.

Peel, seed, and cook vegetables and fruits when possible. Large amounts of raw foods and fiber can be hard to digest when you have SIBO and can increase symptoms. That said, it's important to include fruits and vegetables in your diet—but for easiest digestion, they should be peeled, deseeded, and well cooked (until soft). Get creative by incorporating them into purees, mashes, compotes, soups, and stews. While some people with SIBO can eat raw vegetables, it's helpful to limit them to a side salad or a few raw items and take note of any symptoms. If you are seeing undigested food in your stool, your body is likely having a hard time with digestion.

Be mindful of hard-to-digest foods. In the beginning, you'll want to avoid consuming large amounts of hard-to-digest items like nuts or coconut. Also, be conscious of whether alcohol or caffeine is causing issues and should be removed from your diet.

When possible, avoid snacking between meals. The MMC (see page 5) performs a cleaning wave of the small intestine when caloric intake is suspended for four or five hours, such as between meals. For some people with malabsorption and unintended weight loss, leaving this much time between meals isn't possible. In that case, try to leave some time between meals and lengthen that window over time, as long as it doesn't bring on feelings of dizziness, headaches, and so on.

Seek medical help when you need it. If you are following a SIBO diet and still having unmanageable symptoms, find a physician and/or nutritionist who can support you. Some people will have additional issues, such as fat malabsorption, fructose malabsorption, food sensitivities, or histamine intolerance. Help is available, so please get that help so you can heal.

SIBO DIET OPTIONS

Choosing a SIBO diet can be confusing. Often, a doctor or nutritionist will recommend a specific diet because they have seen positive results or because it's one with which they are familiar. I recommend doing some basic research on the different diets to see which one will benefit you most. The most restrictive diets are the SIBO Specific Food Guide (SSFG) and the Bi-Phasic diet. Since they are the most restrictive, they also relieve the most symptoms. However, those with moderate to low symptoms may not need a restrictive diet, and restricting oneself more than necessary may cause feelings of deprivation, anger, or depression. Also, those with a history of diagnosed eating disorders or known disordered eating should choose a less restrictive diet when possible. Regardless of which you choose, none of these diets are meant to be long-term. SIBO diets are meant to be used short-term as a way to control symptoms.

Some people will start with a more restrictive diet if they are extremely symptomatic and then will move to a less restrictive diet as they begin to heal. Within each diet, people should eat as wide a variety of food as possible. This will support your microbiome and long-term health. Once an overgrowth is cleared, it's helpful and important to reintroduce high-FODMAP foods that you don't react to back into your diet.

The following are the SIBO diets widely used and recommended by doctors:

Low-FODMAP. The low-FODMAP diet, which is used in this cookbook, removes fermentable carbohydrates that may feed a bacterial overgrowth and cause symptoms. It can include grains and starchy vegetables as tolerated.

Specific Carbohydrate Diet (SCD). SCD has been studied to be effective for those with irritable bowel disease (IBD, which includes Crohn's and ulcerative colitis). It removes all polysaccharides including grains and sugars other than honey. It does not remove high FODMAPs.

Gut and Psychology Syndrome (GAPS) diet. Dr. Natasha Campbell-McBride created this diet based on SCD. She focuses more on juicing and fermented foods.

Cedars-Sinai Low Fermentation diet. This SIBO diet was created by Dr. Mark Pimentel. The diet removes dairy that contains lactose as well as beans, legumes, indigestible sugars such as xylitol, high-fiber grains, and some vegetables. Dr. Pimentel also recommends this diet to avoid relapse of SIBO. This diet does not remove high-FODMAP foods.

SIBO Specific Food Guide (SSFG). SSFG, created by Dr. Allison Siebecker, is a combination of SCD, low-FODMAP, and the doctor's clinical experience. It is more restrictive than other diets but may relieve more symptoms for those who are extremely symptomatic.

Bi-phasic diet. The Bi-Phasic diet, by Dr. Nirala Jacobi, is based on SSFG and the doctor's clinical experience. This two-phase diet is more restrictive in the beginning and broadens over time.

Foods to Avoid, Eat in Moderation, and Eat Freely on a SIBO Diet

Although some foods may be in the Foods to Eat in Moderation or Foods to Eat Freely columns in the following table, they may still not be tolerated by all individuals. Some people have issues with raw, rough, or higher-fiber foods or starchier items categorized as low-FODMAP. Likewise, some moderate- and high-FODMAP foods may be tolerated, as not everyone reacts to all high-FODMAP foods. See Resources on page 108 for an app that provides greater detail and specific food brands, is continually updated, and gives specific amounts for each food.

FOODS TO AVOID	FOODS TO EAT IN MODERATION	FOODS TO EAT FREELY*
BEVERAGES Alcohol: high-sugar dessert wines, rum Fruit juices: apple juice Teas: chamomile, fennel, and oolong **GRAINS** Breads: naan or roti, oatmeal, pumpernickel, rye, and mutli-grain wheat bread Flours: amaranth, barley, chestnut, coconut, einkorn, kamut, rye, spelt (unsieved), and wheat Grain flakes: barley, spelt	**BEVERAGES** Alcohol: beer, gin, vodka, whiskey, and wine (except for high-sugar dessert wines) Cocoa powder (for hot chocolate) Coffee Fruit juices: coconut water, cranberry juice, freshly squeezed orange juice Kombucha tea Teas: black, green, peppermint, rooibos, and white **DAIRY** Cheese Coconut yogurt Lactose-free milk Non-dairy milks including almond, coconut, oat, and quinoa	**DAIRY** 24-hour (lactose-free) yogurt Butter **FATS AND OILS** Avocado oil, canola oil, coconut oil, duck fat, garlic-infused oil, olive oil, peanut oil, rice bran oil, sesame oil, sunflower oil, truffle oil, vegetable oil, and walnut oil **GRAINS** Flours: corn (masa harina), millet, quinoa, rice, sorghum, spelt flour (sieved), and teff flour Starches: arrowroot, potato, and tapioca Hominy (canned), drained Nutritional yeast flakes Rice: basmati, brown, white

*All of these foods are low or no FODMAP foods. There are some items some people will not tolerate, specifically some of the flours and starches.

FOODS TO AVOID	FOODS TO EAT IN MODERATION	FOODS TO EAT FREELY*
Grains: couscous, wheat germ, freekeh/farik, rolled oats, fine semolina	**GRAINS** Breads: corn, gluten-free, millet, spelt, white (depending on ingredients), and white sourdough	**MEAT, EGGS, AND FISH** All meats, eggs, and fish unless prepared with high-FODMAP ingredients
LEGUMES Beans: cranberry (borlotti) beans, fava beans, navy beans, kidney beans (boiled), and split peas	Corn tortillas (serving sizes differ for those with and without added gums or fiber)	**NUTS** Peanuts
Tofu (silken)	Flours: almond flour, gluten-free flour, green banana flour	
NUTS Cashews (if not soaked), pistachios	Grains: amaranth (puffed), barley (pearl), buckwheat flakes, bulgur, bran (oat, rice, and wheat; see app for details), buckwheat, millet (hulled), polenta, quick oats or oat groats, quinoa, red rice	
	Starches including corn	
	LEGUMES Beans: black beans, butter beans, chickpeas (canned), lentils, pinto beans	
	Tempeh	
	Tofu, regular or firm (drained)	

*All of these foods are low or no FODMAP foods. There are some items some people will not tolerate, specifically some of the flours and starches.

CONTINUED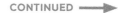

FOODS TO AVOID	FOODS TO EAT IN MODERATION	FOODS TO EAT FREELY*
VEGETABLES AND FRUIT Fruits: apricots (dried), peaches (clingstone) Vegetables: ancho chile, black garlic, button mushrooms, cauliflower, chipotle chile, garlic, Jerusalem artichokes, red and white onions, and shallots	**NUTS AND SEEDS** Nuts: almonds, Brazil nuts, cashews (soaked), chestnuts, hazelnuts, macadamia nuts, pecans, pine nuts, tigernuts, and walnuts Seeds: chia, flax, hemp, poppy, pumpkin, sesame, and sunflower seeds **VEGETABLES AND FRUIT** Fruits: avocado, banana, blueberries, cantaloupe, cherries, coconut, cranberries, dates, honeydew melon, guava (unripe), kiwifruit, lemon, lime, mango, persimmon, pineapple, raspberries Vegetables: alfalfa sprouts, artichokes (globe, fresh or canned), asparagus, beets, bitter melon, bok choy, broccoli, broccolini, Brussels sprouts, butternut squash, cabbage, cassava, celeriac, celery, chicory leaves, corn (canned or fresh), dulse flakes, edamame, eggplant, fennel, green beans, green bell pepper, jicama, kohlrabi, leeks, oyster mushrooms, peas, scallions (green parts only), spaghetti squash, sweet potato, rutabaga, tomatoes (cherry, Roma), zucchini	**VEGETABLES AND FRUIT** Fruits: clementines, grapes (red or green), guava (ripe), oranges, papaya, rhubarb, and strawberries Vegetables: arugula, bamboo shoots, bean sprouts, carrots, collard greens, cucumber, endive, ginger, kabocha squash, kale, lettuce (butter, iceberg, red), olives (black and green), parsnips, potatoes, radishes, red bell peppers, Swiss chard, tomatoes (common)

*All of these foods are low or no FODMAP foods. There are some items some people will not tolerate, specifically some of the flours and starches.

Setting Up Your Healing Kitchen

In this section, we will remove foods that may cause SIBO symptoms, and we'll replace them with staples that will set you up for success. We'll tackle this in three parts: your pantry, fridge, and freezer. Once you've restocked your food, we'll explore equipment that is helpful for the recipes in this book. A little reorganizing means you won't need to scramble every time you want to make something to eat. You'll be ready to create 30-minute meals that support your health and energy every day.

The 30-Minute Pantry

Remove:

× High-fiber grains and whole wheat bread

× Onions and garlic

× Tomato sauce with garlic or onion

× Processed food with high-FODMAP ingredients such as onion or garlic, dried fruit, and spice mixtures that include onion or garlic

Replace:

▶ Garlic cloves with garlic oil

▶ High-fiber grains with white rice, white rice noodles, or fresh vegetable noodles

Add the following pantry staples:

✓ Oils such as avocado, coconut, garlic, ghee, and/or olive oil

✓ Spices such as cinnamon, cumin, Italian seasoning without added garlic, nutmeg, pepper, and sea salt

✓ Pantry vegetables such as squash, sweet potatoes, and white potatoes

✓ Low-FODMAP vegetable stock (see Resources on page 108, for details)

✓ Coconut milk without gums

✓ Sweeteners like honey, maple syrup, or whole cane sugar

✓ Grains such as white rice and white rice noodles

✓ Nut butters that contain only nuts and salt

The 30-Minute Fridge

Remove:

✕ Processed foods with high-FODMAP ingredients, such as lunch meats

✕ Sausages with high-FODMAP ingredients

✕ Cauliflower

✕ Button mushrooms

✕ Salad dressings and other condiments with high-FODMAP ingredients

Replace:

▶ Regular yogurt with homemade or store-bought (see Resources on page 108) yogurt that has been fermented for 24 hours (24-hour yogurt is lactose free and has high levels of probiotics)

▶ Onions or shallots with scallions or chives

▶ Regular dairy milk with lactose-free milk or almond, oat, or rice milk

Add the following refrigerator staples:

✓ Vegetables such as broccoli, carrots, eggplant, parsnips, scallions (green part), spinach, and zucchini

✓ Low-FODMAP mayonnaise, mustard, and other condiments

✓ Fresh fruits such as blueberries, kiwifruit, lemons, limes, oranges, and strawberries

✓ Fresh wild-caught fish

- ✓ Free-range and organic beef or chicken, including cooked rotisserie chicken

- ✓ Bacon or prosciutto

- ✓ Organic butter from free-range cows

- ✓ Organic eggs from free-range chickens

- ✓ Lactose-free cheese (the nutrition label will read 0 sugars; see Resources on page 108, for information about a low-FODMAP app that provides specifics)

- ✓ Fresh herbs such as basil, cilantro, mint, parsley, and rosemary

- ✓ Purchased or premade cooked rice (as tolerated)

The 30-Minute Freezer

Remove and replace processed frozen foods containing high-FODMAP ingredients, including ice cream and packaged frozen meals. Replace high-FODMAP broths with low-FODMAP frozen broths. Here are some freezer staples you'll want to have in low-FODMAP varieties:

- ▸ Frozen beef, chicken, or vegetable broths

- ▸ Frozen bananas, blueberries, raspberries, and strawberries

- ▸ Frozen homemade soups

- ▸ Frozen homemade meals

- ▸ Premade frozen smoothie packets including items such as frozen bananas, frozen spinach, and/or frozen milk (can be made in ice cube trays)

Another freezer note: The recipes in this book all take 30 minutes or less to prepare, but even so, some days it's nice to not have to prepare a meal. When you find a recipe you like that will freeze well, double or triple it, and freeze it in individual portions. Making and freezing large batches of chicken, beef, or vegetable broth can also make things easier when it comes time to make soups. When you are feeling more energetic, you can take time to stock the freezer with items to support you on the days when you'd like a ready-made meal solution.

Multitasking Cooking Equipment

Just a few basic tools are used in multiple recipes and make prep and cooking more efficient. Here are some that I keep handy in my kitchen:

Food processor. This time-saver is used in a variety of recipes in this book.

Chef's knife. A good-quality chef's knife can make cooking enjoyable and prep a breeze. If you're new to cooking, consider taking a knife-skills class or watching online videos to sharpen your skills.

Medium/large skillet. A skillet is essential for sautéing vegetables and more.

Medium to large saucepan or Dutch oven. A saucepan is indispensable for making soups and sauces.

Baking sheets. Baking sheets are key for roasting vegetables and other foods.

Blender, hand mixer, and/or immersion blender. I use a blender to make smoothies and sauces, a hand mixer with a whisk attachment for making mashed potatoes and baked items, and an immersion blender for blending compotes and soups.

THE 30-MINUTE SHOPPING TRIP: A GROCERY LIST

One easy thing about the SIBO diet is that most grocery shopping is done around the perimeter of the market. That's because you'll be purchasing less processed food and focusing more on fresh fruits and vegetables, meats, fish, and fresh herbs. You will have to detour down a few aisles to get healthy oils, spices, white rice, white rice noodles, and a couple of canned or jarred low-FODMAP foods.

Your exact grocery list will depend on the recipes you choose, but here's an example of some items you might need.

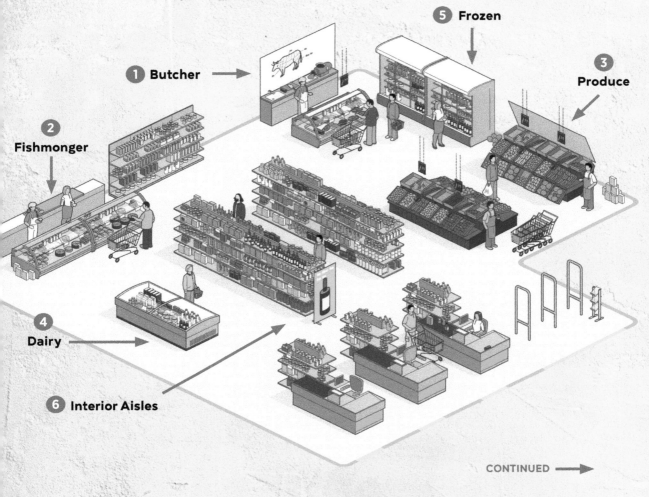

5 Frozen

1 Butcher

3 Produce

2 Fishmonger

4 Dairy

6 Interior Aisles

CONTINUED →

Butcher 1 and fishmonger 2

☐ Free-range and organic beef or chicken

☐ Fresh wild-caught fish

Produce 3

☐ Bananas (1 bunch)
☐ Basil (1 bunch)
☐ Blueberries (1 pint)
☐ Broccoli (1 pound)
☐ Carrots (1 pound)
☐ Cilantro (1 bunch)
☐ Eggplant (1 pound)
☐ Kiwifruit (6)
☐ Lemons (6)
☐ Limes (6)
☐ Mint (1 bunch)

☐ Oranges (3)
☐ Parsley (1 bunch)
☐ Parsnips (1 pound)
☐ Rosemary (1 bunch)
☐ Scallions (1 bunch)
☐ Spinach (1 bunch)
☐ Squash (1 pound)
☐ Strawberries (1 pint)
☐ Sweet potatoes (1 pound)
☐ White potatoes (1 pound)
☐ Zucchini (1 pound)

Dairy 4

☐ 24-hour yogurt (1 jar)
☐ Organic butter from free-range cows (1 pound)

☐ Lactose-free cheese (the nutrition label will read 0 sugars; see Resources on page 108, for low-FODMAP app information)

Frozen 5

☐ Frozen blueberries (1 bag)
☐ Frozen raspberries (1 bag)

☐ Frozen strawberries (1 bag)

Interior aisles 6

- ☐ Aluminum foil and parchment paper
- ☐ Canned coconut milk without gums (2 cans)
- ☐ Ghee and oils such as avocado, coconut, garlic, and olive oil (1 bottle each)
- ☐ Grains such as white rice and white rice noodles (1 bag each)
- ☐ Low-FODMAP mayonnaise and mustard (1 jar each)
- ☐ Nut butters such as almond butter, with only the ingredients almonds and salt (1 jar)
- ☐ Organic eggs from free-range chickens (1 dozen)
- ☐ Spices such as black pepper, cinnamon, cumin, Italian seasoning (without garlic), nutmeg, and salt (1 jar each)
- ☐ Sweeteners like honey, maple syrup, and whole cane sugar (1 package each)

When You're the Only One in Your Household on a Restrictive Diet

Many people with SIBO live with family members who are not on a restricted diet. This cookbook is geared to making quick and easy meals that most everyone will appreciate. If you're serving a dish to someone who isn't on a SIBO diet, you can offer an additional processed carbohydrate such as dinner rolls, tortillas, or bread with the meal you're making for yourself. It can also be helpful to make a family-style dish, where everyone can pick their own add-ons.

At times, you may be making something that doesn't appeal to others in your home. In that case, you can pick another easy meal to cook for other family members or declare that it's a "leftovers" or "do it yourself" night!

About the Recipes

The recipes in this book are designed to be quick, straightforward, and flavorful. They will help you get to know the different low-FODMAP ingredients as well as ways to incorporate them into various dishes.

The 30-Minute Promise

The 30-minute promise means 30 minutes—all in. No extra time for chopping, simmering, or slow cooking. This book exclusively features fresh and simple recipes that can be made in 30 minutes or less. Sometimes you'll be able to utilize convenience items to make preparation even quicker.

I recommend buying organic meats and wild-caught fish whenever possible because meat and fish are more likely to contain toxins if they are not raised in humane environments. For fruits and vegetables, buy organic whenever possible, but to make the most of your organic dollar, consult the Dirty Dozen and Clean Fifteen (see Resources on page 108) to learn which types of produce contain more or fewer pesticide residues.

About the Labels and Tips

All the recipes in this book fall within the low-FODMAP diet. Some recipes will include multiple options for a certain ingredient, such as using either honey or maple syrup.

In addition to being low-FODMAP, each recipe will also identify which other diets it fits under, including SCD, GAPS, Cedars-Sinai, SSFG, or Bi-phasic.

With these labels, readers on any of these diets will be able to use this cookbook and easily see which recipes will work for them. Each recipe will be color-coded as follows: (BPD) BPD—Bi-Phasic diet, (CSD) CSD—Cedars-Sinai diet, (GAPS) GAPS—Gut and Psychology Syndrome diet, (LFD) LFD—Low-FODMAP diet, (SCD) SCD—Specific Carbohydrate diet, and (SSFG) SSFG—SIBO Specific Food Guide.

The recipes are also labeled if they are dairy-free, egg-free, gluten-free, nut-free, and/or vegetarian. Each recipe is followed by a helpful tip:

SIBO tip. Highlights important SIBO issues in conjunction with the recipe.

Make it easier. Provides ways to cut down on effort, such as using dried herbs instead of chopped or buying pre-chopped vegetables.

Ingredient swaps. Swaps in new ingredients that may make the dish take on another flavor profile.

Speed it up. Speeds up the already-quick process.

Learning More Can Empower You

When I started a SIBO diet, I had to adapt to a new way of thinking and cooking. I had to make sure that I had the right ingredients and some pre-pared food on hand so I wasn't stuck without a meal when I was tired or sick. And I had to (slowly!) understand which foods I tolerated and which ones I didn't. It was a steep learning curve for me at the time, but a lot was different then. Now that we know more, I want to make the learning curve easier for you. By exploring and testing these recipes, you'll begin to understand what foods work for you, learn easy cooking methods, and see how delicious food can be on a SIBO diet. Many of my clients remark that they've learned a great deal about nutrition and their health. I hope that comes to be true for you, too.

LIFE BEYOND YOUR KITCHEN

No one should be on a SIBO diet long-term, but some people may need to make some permanent changes to their diets. For instance, I no longer eat gluten, and I eat minimal dairy. When I had SIBO, I couldn't tolerate eggs, but now I'm fine with them. Depending on your underlying cause of SIBO and any concurrent health issues, relapse can be common. Adding in high-FODMAP foods over time while also revisiting your food tolerances regularly will help you stay healthy. As you begin your new diet, here are some things to remember:

Meal prep when possible. Double a recipe and freeze some for later, prep lunches ahead of time, or enlist a family member to help you with meals.

Look at social gatherings in a new way. Bring something that you know you can eat if you're attending a cocktail party. Communicate with the host about it in advance. Having people over for dinner at your home where you control the meal ingredients may be easier. And it's okay to say no to some invitations in order to prioritize your health if you're not feeling well.

Find your special restaurant. Look for a restaurant or two where you can review the menu in advance or speak with the chef about your dietary needs. A smart place to start is to order a protein with only salt and pepper (no marinades), vegetables, and rice or other starch as tolerated, cooked and seasoned with just salt and pepper and your oil of choice. Over time, hopefully you'll find your special place where you know the chef and can always count on a good meal that works for you.

Alcohol doesn't work for many people who have SIBO. Others are able to have small amounts of wine (see Resources on page 108) or other low-FODMAP beverages. If you decide to drink, do so slowly and check in with how you feel.

Book a vacation rental with a kitchen. When planning a vacation, consider renting a space with a kitchen so you can eat some meals at home. Research restaurants and grocery stores ahead of time. Additionally, if you plan some 30-minute meals from this cookbook in advance, you'll spend less time cooking and more time vacationing!

Reset Your Gut and Enjoy Your Life

Healing from SIBO isn't always a straight line. There may be times when you want to give up, go off your diet, and never talk about SIBO again! You may feel like you're not getting better even though you're doing everything in your power to do so. These are very normal and common feelings. If you eat off your diet because you're feeling deprived, pay attention to how the food makes you feel. Either it will give you information that you can use to widen your diet, or it will give you symptoms that reassure you that being on a SIBO diet is the most helpful choice right now.

Often, when symptoms go away, we forget them and instead focus on other things that are wrong. If you keep a food and symptom diary, reviewing it may surprise you and show you that you are indeed healing. If that's not true for you, check in with your health care provider. Do you feel like they are invested in your case and know about SIBO? Do you need additional resources? You may benefit from seeing multiple practitioners including a doctor, body worker, nutritionist, and/or therapist. See what feels right for you and check in with yourself often.

You Can Do This, 30 Minutes at a Time

By reading this chapter, you've taken a big step in your healing journey. Change can feel overwhelming, but breaking it into bite-size pieces can make it much more manageable. That's why all of these recipes can be made in 30 minutes or less. The goal here is to make cooking simpler and more enjoyable. During this time, it's also important to lighten your schedule if you can and take time to relieve stress in ways that work for you. Even when you may be feeling not so great, it doesn't mean you can't experience joy. Actively practice gratitude, seek out those who can support you during this time, be there for others when possible, practice being in the present moment, and enjoy the fullness of your life, with all its peaks and valleys. Now, on to the recipes—bon appétit, and cheers to your health and healing!

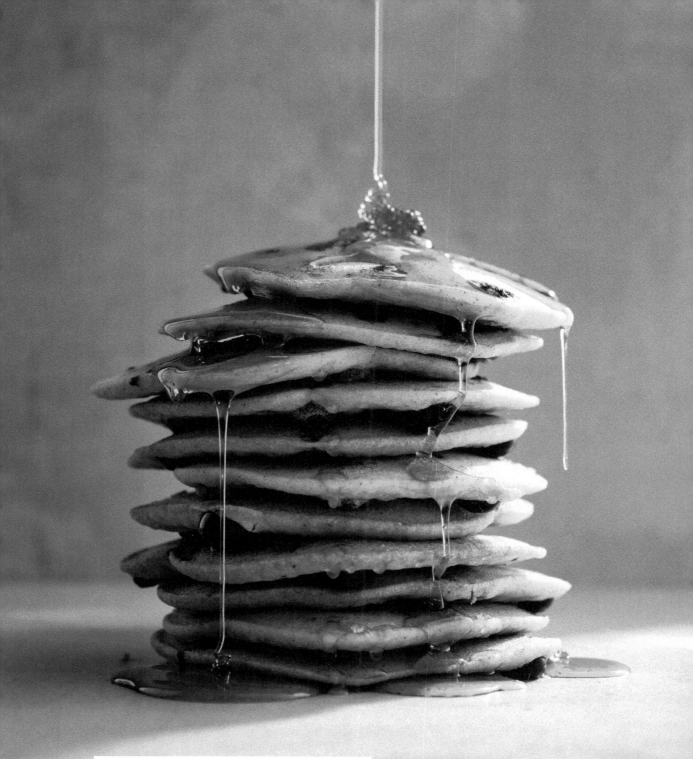

Cinnamon-Blueberry Rice Flour Pancakes, page 30

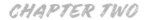

CHAPTER TWO

Quick Breakfasts

Breakfast is considered the most important meal of the day. But for many of us, it's challenging to get breakfast together as we're getting ready for a busy workday. This chapter focuses on quick, delicious breakfasts that can be made in advance or made quickly in the morning. I love the Pumpkin Smoothie Bowl (page 27) for a nutritious, filling cool treat. The Strawberry Rhubarb Compote (page 26) is both tangy and sweet and can be served warm alongside the egg dishes in this chapter or cold with 24-hour yogurt.

Strawberry Rhubarb Compote

Compotes are a great way to add cooked fruit to your diet. This compote combines the sweetness of strawberries and the tartness of rhubarb for a classically delicious taste. Enjoy this warm or cold, on pancakes, with 24-hour yogurt, or over warm rice cereal. It's important to buy organic strawberries since strawberries have the highest amount of pesticide residue of all conventionally raised produce.

Serves 6 (½-cup servings)
Prep time: 5 minutes
Cook time: 20 minutes

2 tablespoons butter or coconut oil
4 large rhubarb stalks, cut into 1-inch pieces
1 pound frozen organic strawberries
6 tablespoons whole cane sugar or honey (use sugar for (LFD); use honey for (BPD), (GAPS), (SCD), or (SSFG))
Grated zest from 1 large orange

1. In a medium saucepan over medium heat, combine the butter, rhubarb, strawberries, sugar, and orange zest. Bring the mixture to a simmer.

2. Simmer for about 15 minutes, breaking the fruit apart with a spoon as it begins to break down and thicken.

3. Remove the compote from the heat. Serve the compote immediately by itself, or let it cool slightly and serve it with your side of choice.

SIBO tip: A research study on women 70 years and older showed less cognitive loss in those who consumed at least 1 to 2 servings of strawberries per week. Rhubarb doesn't contain any FODMAPs, so it can be eaten in any amount.

Per serving (½ cup): Calories: 111; Total fat: 4g; Saturated fat: 3g; Cholesterol: 10mg; Sodium: 33mg; Carbohydrates: 20g; Sugar: 16g; Fiber: 2g; Protein: 1g

Pumpkin Smoothie Bowl

Smoothies are great for some people with SIBO because they provide additional hydration via their liquid content and they're an easy breakfast option. If you don't seem to tolerate a smoothie with raw foods, try one (like this one!) that contains some cooked vegetables. Top this bowl with coconut flakes, pumpkin seeds, pecan pieces, or dairy-free chocolate chips!

Serves 2

Prep time: 10 minutes

⅔ cup pumpkin puree

8 ice cubes

½ cup 24-hour yogurt or low-FODMAP non-dairy yogurt

½ cup brewed coffee or espresso, cold or at room temperature

¼ cup coconut cream

2 tablespoons maple syrup or honey (use maple syrup for (LFD); use honey for (BPD), (GAPS), (SCD), or (SSFG))

1 tablespoon pumpkin pie spice

2 medium frozen bananas (unripe for (LFD); ripe for (BPD), (GAPS), (SCD), or (SSFG))

2 tablespoons collagen powder (optional, for added protein)

1. In a blender, combine the pumpkin puree, ice cubes, yogurt, coffee, coconut cream, syrup, pumpkin pie spice, bananas, and collagen powder (if using).

2. Blend for 1 minute or until fully blended.

3. Divide into two bowls and add the toppings of your choice. Serve immediately.

Ingredient swap: Feel free to add more cooked vegetables to your smoothies. For greens like spinach, simply sauté the spinach and then divide it into an ice cube tray. Cover it with low-FODMAP milk if you choose, freeze it, and *voilà*— portioned ingredients you can throw into a smoothie anytime!

Per serving: Calories: 293; Total fat: 9g; Saturated fat: 8g; Cholesterol: 6mg; Sodium: 34mg; Carbohydrates: 51g; Sugar: 31g; Fiber: 5g; Protein: 4g

Fruit & Yogurt Jar

This versatile dish can be made in advance for a quick breakfast on the go. You can also create a yogurt jar using nut butter or compote if desired. When starting a SIBO diet, it's recommended to first try cooked fruit before moving on to raw fruit.

Serves 4

Prep time: 15 minutes

2 cups plain 24-hour yogurt or low-FODMAP non-dairy yogurt

2 tablespoons maple syrup or honey (use maple syrup for low-FODMAP; use honey for (BPD), (GAPS), (SCD), or (SSFG))

1 medium banana, sliced (ripe for (BPD), (GAPS), (SCD), or (SSFG))

2 kiwifruit, cut into small chunks

1 cup blueberries

½ cup Nutty Cinnamon Granola (page 29, optional)

1. In a medium bowl, whisk together the yogurt and sweetener. Set aside.

2. Place the banana slices on the bottom of four half-pint Mason jars. Spoon ½ cup of the yogurt mixture into each jar. Place the kiwifruit on top of the yogurt, add a layer of blueberries, and top with the granola (if using).

3. Enjoy immediately or store in the refrigerator for up to 2 days.

Ingredient tip: It's always important to "eat the rainbow," and fruit can be an enjoyable part of that. Kiwifruit is an excellent source of vitamins C and K. Nutrient-dense blueberries have anti-inflammatory and antioxidant properties and have been shown to lower blood pressure.

Per serving: Calories: 164; Total fat: 4g; Saturated fat: 3g; Cholesterol: 13mg; Sodium: 33mg; Carbohydrates: 28g; Sugar: 19g; Fiber: 3g; Protein: 5g

Nutty Cinnamon Granola

If you're missing breakfast cereal, try granola! Grocery-store cereals are fortified with nutrients, but those nutrients don't come from whole foods. Homemade granola offers a healthier yet still delicious SIBO-friendly option.

Serves 5 (½-cup servings)
Prep time: 5 minutes
Cook time: 25 minutes

½ cup large unsweetened coconut flakes
½ cup raw slivered or chopped almonds
½ cup raw pecan pieces
½ cup raw walnut pieces
¼ cup raw pumpkin seeds
¼ cup raw sunflower seeds
¼ cup dried cranberries
⅛ cup chia seeds (omit for
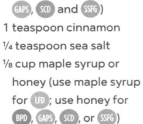 GAPS, SCD and SSFG)
1 teaspoon cinnamon
¼ teaspoon sea salt
⅛ cup maple syrup or honey (use maple syrup for LFD ; use honey for BPD, GAPS, SCD, or SSFG)
1 tablespoon melted coconut oil
1 teaspoon vanilla extract

1. Preheat the oven to 350°F. Line a baking sheet with aluminum foil or parchment paper.

2. In a large bowl, combine the coconut flakes, almonds, pecans, walnuts, pumpkin seeds, sunflower seeds, dried cranberries, chia seeds, cinnamon, salt, sweetener, oil, and vanilla. Mix together well and spread the mixture onto the lined baking sheet.

3. Bake the granola for 8 minutes, stir, and bake for another 8 minutes. Remove from the oven and let cool for about 7 minutes on a baking rack.

4. Serve immediately in a bowl with your milk of choice, or cool completely and store in a sealed container at room temperature for up to 3 weeks.

SIBO tip: Nuts can be hard to digest. To determine your tolerance, first try nut milk, then nut butter, and then whole nuts. Chewing your food until it becomes liquid in your mouth before you swallow can support digestion. Some people also find it helpful to take a digestive enzyme before meals.

Per serving: Calories: 474; Total fat: 40g; Saturated fat: 12g; Cholesterol: 0mg; Sodium: 125mg; Carbohydrates: 25g; Sugar: 13g; Fiber: 9g; Protein: 10g

Cinnamon-Blueberry Rice Flour Pancakes

Pancakes are something people don't have to miss when they go on a SIBO diet. Not everyone will tolerate gluten-free flour since it often contains gums. These pancakes are made with rice flour to avoid this problem.

Serves 4

Prep time: 5 minutes

Cook time: 15 minutes

2 cups rice flour

2 teaspoons baking powder

1 teaspoon cinnamon

½ teaspoon sea salt

2 tablespoons maple syrup

2 large eggs, slightly beaten

1½ cups low-FODMAP milk of choice, divided

2 teaspoons avocado oil

1 teaspoon vanilla extract

1 cup fresh or frozen blueberries

4 teaspoons ghee, avocado oil, or coconut oil, divided

1. In a medium bowl, mix together the rice flour, baking powder, cinnamon, and salt. Add the maple syrup, eggs, 1¼ cups of milk, avocado oil, and vanilla. Mix until incorporated. Stir in up to ¼ cup additional milk if the batter is too thick. Gently stir in the blueberries.

2. Heat a large skillet over medium-high heat. Add 1 teaspoon of ghee. Swirl the ghee in the pan and then pour ¼-cup scoops of batter into the pan to make three (3- to 4-inch) pancakes.

3. Cook for 2 to 3 minutes or until bubbles appear on top of the pancakes. Flip the pancakes and let them cook on the other side for another 2 minutes. Remove the pancakes from the pan and repeat for the remaining batches, adding 1 teaspoon more ghee before each batch. Serve immediately. Pancakes can be refrigerated for up to 5 days or frozen for 3 months.

SIBO tip: Rice flour and cooled cooked rice have resistant starch, which is starch that is resistant to digestion, similar to soluble fiber. If you tolerate freshly cooked rice but not rice flour or rewarmed rice, you may be sensitive to resistant starch.

Per serving: Calories: 452; Total fat: 11g; Saturated fat: 4g; Cholesterol: 104mg; Sodium: 633mg; Carbohydrates: 77g; Sugar: 10g; Fiber: 3g; Protein: 9g

The Best Hard-Boiled Eggs

If you've been avoiding boiling eggs because it sounds difficult or your eggs never come out right, try this recipe. I like to hard-boil eggs over the weekend for the week ahead. They are great over salads, in bowls, as egg salad (see page 46), or halved with some sea salt and low-FODMAP hot sauce (as tolerated).

Serves 4

Cook time: 30 minutes

8 large eggs

1. Fill a large saucepan with about 4 inches of water. The pot should be big enough so all the eggs can sit in the saucepan in a single layer.

2. Over high heat, bring the water to a boil. Gently lower the eggs four at a time into the boiling water using a spiral wire skimmer. Boil for 30 seconds. Reduce the heat to a low simmer, cover, and simmer for 13 minutes.

3. Meanwhile, fill a medium bowl with two trays of ice cubes and water to cover the ice cubes. Gently lower the eggs into the ice water. Let cool for 10 minutes.

4. Tap each egg against the counter on opposite sides of the egg. Then gently roll the egg against the counter while you feel the shell cracking. Remove the eggshell; it should come off very easily. Serve immediately.

5. Cover leftover peeled eggs with a damp paper towel, place them in a resealable container, and store them in the refrigerator for up to 7 days.

Per serving: Calories: 155; Total fat: 11g; Saturated fat: 3g; Cholesterol: 373mg; Sodium: 124mg; Carbohydrates: 1g; Sugar: 1g; Fiber: 0g; Protein: 13g

Creamy Herb-Scrambled Eggs

Chives are sometimes mistaken for scallions or green onions (which are the same thing), but they are slenderer than scallions and look a bit like hollow grass. They complement many dishes, including eggs, baked potatoes, and soups. Parsley contains antioxidants and volatile oils, which have been shown to inhibit tumor formation in the lungs. Parsley is also a good source of vitamin C and folate for heart health. We'll use both herbs in this tasty egg dish.

Serves 4

Prep time: 5 minutes

Cook time: 20 minutes

9 large eggs

¼ cup low-FODMAP milk

¼ cup ghee, butter, or avocado oil

¼ cup freshly grated Parmesan cheese

2 tablespoons chopped fresh parsley

1 tablespoon chopped fresh chives

½ teaspoon sea salt

¼ teaspoon freshly ground black pepper

½ lemon, cut into four wedges

1. Crack the eggs into a medium bowl and then add the milk. Whisk for 1 minute.

2. In a medium skillet over medium-low heat, melt the ghee. Pour the egg mixture into the pan and stir the eggs with a spatula until they begin to look creamy. Immediately add the Parmesan cheese, parsley, chives, salt, and pepper, continuing to stir.

3. Once the eggs are cooked but still look moist, remove them from the heat and divide them among four plates. Squeeze one lemon wedge over the eggs on each plate. Serve immediately.

Speed it up: Cooking eggs at a low temperature makes them creamy and custardy. But if you're in a hurry, turn the temperature up to medium. You'll still get some of that creaminess but quicker.

Per serving: Calories: 319; Total fat: 27g; Saturated fat: 13g; Cholesterol: 457mg; Sodium: 527mg; Carbohydrates: 2g; Sugar: 2g; Fiber: <1g; Protein: 17g

GLUTEN-FREE | NUT-FREE | VEGETARIAN
DIETS: CSD, LFD

Fried Egg & Avocado on Sweet Potato Toast

Here's a nutritious new way to do toast! We'll add an egg and avocado for a balanced meal in just 15 minutes. Pick a sweet potato that is large and tube-shaped so you can get more slices out of the middle of it. Half a cup of sweet potatoes is considered low-FODMAP.

Serves 4 (1-slice servings)
Prep time: 5 minutes
Cook time: 10 minutes

1 large orange-fleshed
   sweet potato
1 tablespoon ghee, butter,
   or preferred oil
4 large eggs
Sea salt
Freshly ground
   black pepper
½ avocado, cut into
   four slices

1. Peel the sweet potato and cut four (¼-inch) lengthwise slices from the middle of the sweet potato. Place the slices in the toaster on high and cook for one cycle. Check the sweet potato and remove if it is soft and slightly crispy. If not, cook it for one more cycle. Remove and cool for 3 minutes.

2. Meanwhile, place a large skillet over medium-high heat, and melt the ghee. Working in batches if necessary, crack each egg into a separate spot in the pan. Cook for 3 minutes, sprinkling with salt and pepper as desired. Remove the pan from the heat.

3. With a fork, flatten 1 slice of avocado across each slice of sweet potato toast and top with a fried egg. Serve immediately.

Make it easier: Cook some sweet potato slices in the oven at 350°F until they are soft. When you're ready to eat a slice, pop it in the toaster. It will crisp up more quickly because it's already cooked.

Per serving: Calories: 178; Total fat: 11g; Saturated fat: 4g; Cholesterol: 195mg; Sodium: 92mg; Carbohydrates: 12g; Sugar: 3g; Fiber: 3g; Protein: 7g

Bacon Veggie Hash with Eggs

This delicious hash incorporates healthy fats, carbohydrates, and protein. If you prefer soft-cooked eggs over sunny-side up, just add two tablespoons of water to the skillet prior to covering the pan in step 4. This will steam the eggs.

Serves 4

Prep time: 15 minutes

Cook time: 10 minutes

1 teaspoon avocado oil

4 slices bacon, chopped

3 scallions, chopped (green parts only)

2 medium organic russet potatoes

2 large carrots

1 teaspoon Italian seasoning

1 teaspoon sea salt

½ teaspoon freshly ground black pepper

4 large eggs

1. In a large skillet over medium heat, add the oil, bacon, and scallions. Cook for about 4 minutes until the bacon is crispy and the onions are cooked.

2. Meanwhile, peel and then shred the potatoes and carrots using a food processor or grater.

3. When the bacon is crispy, drain the excess grease, leaving about 1 tablespoon in the pan. Add the shredded potatoes and carrots, Italian seasoning, salt, and pepper to the pan.

4. Increase the heat to medium-high and sauté for about 6 minutes or until the vegetables are soft. Using a spoon, create four indentations in the hash. Crack an egg into each indentation. Cover and cook for about 2 minutes until the eggs are cooked to sunny-side up. The whites will be cooked, and the yolks will be wobbly. Divide the hash onto four plates and serve immediately.

SIBO tip: If you've removed grains and starchy vegetables from your diet and are looking to add some back in, try white rice and peeled white potatoes. Since they're high-glycemic, they are unlikely to ferment and feed a bacterial overgrowth. Most people who don't tolerate them will experience a reaction within an hour or two.

Per serving: Calories: 228; Total fat: 10g; Saturated fat: 3g; Cholesterol: 194mg; Sodium: 813mg; Carbohydrates: 24g; Sugar: 3g; Fiber: 3g; Protein: 12g

Cozy Cardamom Honey Latte

Many of my clients ask if they can still drink coffee. It really depends on how you react to coffee. If coffee is hard on your stomach, try decaf. Drinking coffee with milk in the form of a latte can also make it easier on your stomach. This cardamom honey latte may sound fancy, but it's very easy to make.

Serves 4

Prep time: 15 minutes

4 teaspoons honey or maple syrup (use honey for (BPD), (GAPS), (SCD), or (SSFG))

2 teaspoons ground cardamom, divided

4 shots espresso or 2 cups coffee, divided

4 tablespoons collagen powder (optional, for extra protein)

4 cups low-FODMAP milk of choice

1. In each of four coffee cups, place 1 teaspoon of sweetener, ½ teaspoon cardamom, 1 shot espresso or ½ cup coffee, and 1 tablespoon collagen (if using). Mix together.

2. Warm the milk in the microwave for 1 to 2 minutes or in a small saucepan over medium heat for 5 to 7 minutes. Froth it with a hand frother if you have one. Stir in 1 cup of warmed milk into each cup of the cardamom coffee mixture.

3. Enjoy immediately.

SIBO tip: Coffee can be a gut irritant and increase anxiety in some people. If you're not sure whether coffee bothers you, remove it for a week and then reintroduce it. Some people find that decaffeinated coffee works better for them, particularly those prone to anxiety.

Per serving: Calories: 63; Total fat: 3g; Saturated fat: 0g; Cholesterol: 0mg; Sodium: 175mg; Carbohydrates: 8g; Sugar: 6g; Fiber: <1g; Protein: 2g

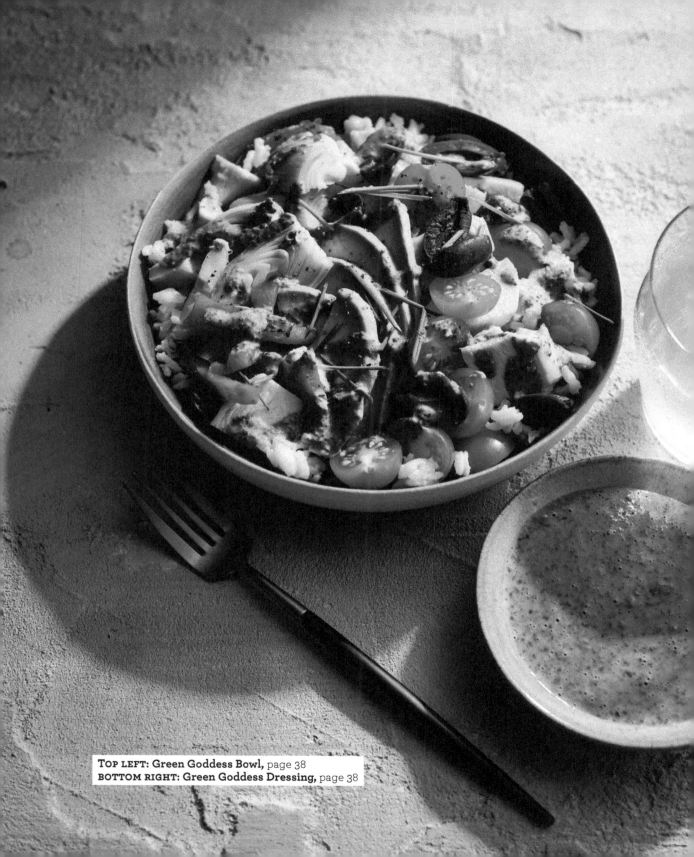

TOP LEFT: Green Goddess Bowl, page 38
BOTTOM RIGHT: Green Goddess Dressing, page 38

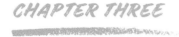
Midday Meals

Lunch refuels us for an energetic and productive afternoon. As part of the 30-minutes-or-less promise, tasty recipes for bowls, salads, wraps, and a delicious chicken noodle soup are offered. Some of these are fresh, and others are made in advance and easily reheated in the lunchroom microwave. My personal favorites are the Curried Chicken Salad (page 45) and the Green Goddess (page 38) and Ginger Beef (page 41) bowls. Both salads and bowls are super versatile and easily portable.

Green Goddess Bowl

Bowls are great to take for lunch because you can prep the ingredients in advance for the week and mix things up using a variety of vegetables, proteins, and dressings for something different each day. Feel free to switch out the vegetables in this bowl You can also switch out the rice for another preferred low-FODMAP grain or starchy vegetable like potatoes, parsnips, or sweet potatoes.

Serves 4

Prep time: 15 minutes

For the Green Goddess Dressing

1 cup parsley leaves

1 cup packed
  spinach leaves

1 cup cilantro leaves

2 tablespoons
  minced chives

3 tablespoons freshly
  squeezed lemon juice

1 tablespoon champagne
  or rice vinegar

¼ cup garlic oil

¼ cup avocado oil

¼ cup low-FODMAP
  mayonnaise

¼ cup 24-hour yogurt
  or low-FODMAP
  dairy-free yogurt

½ teaspoon sea salt

¼ teaspoon freshly ground
  black pepper

To make the Green Goddess Dressing

1. In a blender, combine the parsley, spinach, cilantro, chives, lemon juice, vinegar, garlic oil, avocado oil, mayonnaise, yogurt, salt, and pepper and blend until smooth. Set aside.

For the bowls

4 cups cooked white rice,
    warmed and salted

4 cups cooked rotisserie
    chicken, cubed

½ avocado, sliced

1½ cups halved cherry
    tomatoes

¾ cup kalamata
    olives, halved

¾ cup jarred fire-roasted
    red peppers, chopped
    (without garlic or onion)

1 cup canned, drained
    artichoke hearts,
    quartered

2 tablespoons
    minced chives

To make the bowls

2. Divide the rice among four bowls. Top each bowl with 1 cup chicken, the tomatoes, olives, roasted peppers, and artichoke hearts. Top with 2 tablespoons of dressing (or more as desired) and chives. Serve immediately.

Make it easier: To take this meal on the go, prepare the bowl, but pack the dressing separately. Gently warm the bowl in the microwave for 1 minute and then add the dressing.

Per serving: Calories: 709; Total fat: 38g; Saturated fat: 7g; Cholesterol: 85mg; Sodium: 1469mg; Carbohydrates: 58g; Sugar: 6g; Fiber: 7g; Protein: 34g

DAIRY-FREE | GLUTEN-FREE | NUT-FREE
DIETS: BPD, CSD, LFD

Ground Pork & Veggie Bowl

This bowl makes a delicious dinner but is also great to prep ahead for lunches. Feel free to substitute other vegetables for the scallions, red bell pepper, cabbage, carrots, and water chestnuts.

Serves 4

Prep time: 5 minutes

Cook time: 25 minutes

3 tablespoons avocado
  oil, divided

2 large eggs

1 bunch scallions, chopped
  (green parts only)

1 red bell pepper, chopped

1 pound lean ground pork
  or turkey

¼ cup finely chopped
  fresh ginger

½ teaspoon sea salt

¼ teaspoon freshly ground
  black pepper

1 teaspoon low-FODMAP
  hot sauce (optional)

18 ounces packaged
  coleslaw mix with carrots

¼ cup coconut aminos

2 tablespoons rice vinegar

1 (8-ounce) can sliced
  water chestnuts

1 tablespoon sesame oil

1 tablespoon garlic oil

1. Warm a large skillet over medium-high heat. Heat 1 tablespoon of avocado oil for 1 minute; then add the eggs and mix to scramble. Transfer the eggs onto a small plate and set aside.

2. In the same large skillet over medium-high heat, heat the remaining 2 tablespoons of avocado oil; then add the scallions and bell pepper and sauté for 2 to 3 minutes until soft.

3. Add the pork, ginger, salt, pepper, and hot sauce (if using). Stir and cook until the meat is cooked through, about 10 minutes.

4. Add the coleslaw, coconut aminos, vinegar, water chestnuts, and eggs. Stir and cook until the coleslaw is wilted and tender, about 5 minutes. Remove from the heat and add the sesame and garlic oils. Mix and serve immediately.

5. Store leftovers in the refrigerator for up to 3 days.

Speed it up: Cut some veggies in advance. When you're ready to make a specific meal, you can use your precut vegetables to shorten your prep time.

Per serving: Calories: 418; Total fat: 25g; Saturated fat: 4g; Cholesterol: 160mg; Sodium: 730mg; Carbohydrates: 22g; Sugar: 10g; Fiber: 4g; Protein: 29g

Ginger Beef Bowl

This bowl makes an easy weeknight dinner and tasty leftover lunch. If possible, buy organic, free-range ground beef. If you shop at a farmers' market, you can get to know the purveyors and hear about their animal husbandry practices. Many farms and ranches also offer community-supported agriculture (CSA) meat subscriptions. This can be cheaper and ensure that you are getting the best-quality meat.

Serves 4

Prep time: 15 minutes

Cook time: 15 minutes

2 tablespoons garlic oil

1 bunch scallions, sliced (green parts only), divided

1 red bell pepper, cut into bite-size pieces

1 pound ground beef

⅛ cup fresh minced ginger

3 tablespoons coconut aminos

1 tablespoon honey

1 tablespoon low-FODMAP hot sauce (optional)

4 cups prepared white or brown rice, warmed

¼ cup chopped peanuts or almonds (optional)

1. Warm a large skillet over medium heat. Heat the oil for 30 seconds; then add most of the scallions, reserving 2 tablespoons for later, and the bell pepper, and cook for about 3 minutes until soft.

2. Add the ground beef. Break it up into small pieces and cook until no longer pink, about 8 minutes.

3. Add the ginger, coconut aminos, honey, and hot sauce (if using). Stir until incorporated and cook for 2 minutes. Remove from the heat.

4. Place 1 cup of warm rice in each of four bowls, top with the ground beef mixture, and sprinkle with the remaining scallions and chopped nuts (if using). Enjoy immediately or store in the refrigerator for up to 3 days.

SIBO tip: Since white rice is high-glycemic, it digests quickly, so it's not as likely to feed bacteria as the higher-fiber brown rice.

Per serving: Calories: 532; Total fat: 22g; Saturated fat: 7g; Cholesterol: 70mg; Sodium: 286mg; Carbohydrates: 55g; Sugar: 9g; Fiber: 2g; Protein: 27g

DIETS: BPD, GAPS, LFD, SCD, SSFG

Ranch & Bacon Lettuce Wrap

What's better than salty, crunchy bacon and zesty ranch together? Not much! If you're taking one of these wraps to work, take all the ingredients but assemble the wrap when you're ready to eat.

Serves 4

Prep time: 10 minutes

Cook time: 15 minutes

8 slices bacon

1 cup 24-hour yogurt
or low-FODMAP
non-dairy yogurt

¼ cup grated
Parmesan cheese

1 tablespoon garlic oil

1 tablespoon chopped
fresh chives

1 tablespoon chopped
fresh parsley

1 teaspoon paprika

½ teaspoon sea salt

¼ teaspoon freshly ground
black pepper

16 leaves romaine lettuce

8 slices cheddar cheese
(optional)

2 medium organic
tomatoes, sliced

4 cups rotisserie chicken,
shredded

1. Heat a large heavy skillet over medium heat. Add the bacon slices and cook for about 4 minutes or until the bottom is browned. Flip the bacon and cook for 2 to 3 minutes on the other side until browned. Transfer the bacon to a paper towel.

2. In a small bowl, thoroughly mix the yogurt, Parmesan cheese, oil, chives, parsley, paprika, salt, and pepper. Set aside.

3. Place 4 squares of parchment paper or paper towels on a flat surface. Place 2 pieces of romaine lettuce on each square, facing up, leaving some room on the bottom of the square. Top each pair of lettuce leaves with 2 slices of cheese (if using) and 2 slices of bacon. Divide the tomatoes among the four wraps and place the tomato slices on top of the cheese. Then place 1 cup chicken on top of the tomato slices. Drizzle 2 tablespoons of the prepared ranch dressing on top of the chicken. Place 2 more pieces of romaine on top, facing down.

4. Tuck the bottom of the square against the romaine lettuce and fold the sides over to hold the wrap in place. Enjoy immediately.

Per serving: Calories: 354; Total fat: 16g; Saturated fat: 6g; Cholesterol: 125mg; Sodium: 1058mg; Carbohydrates: 10g; Sugar: 4g; Fiber: 3g; Protein: 43g

Citrus, Shrimp & Rice Salad

I first ate a rice salad when I visited France during my college years. At first, I thought it was so strange that rice would be eaten cold and in a salad! But once I tasted it, I was smitten. Here we'll use citrus to add sweetness, balancing it with savory herbs and vinegar.

Serves 4

Prep time: 10 minutes

½ cup extra-virgin olive oil
Grated zest of
  1 organic orange
3 tablespoons freshly
  squeezed orange juice
2 tablespoons freshly
  squeezed lemon juice
1 tablespoon honey
¼ teaspoon sea salt
1 navel orange, peeled and
  cut into circular slices
1 tangerine or clementine,
  peeled and cut into
  circular slices
4 cups cooked white
  rice, cold
¼ cup chopped fresh
  mint leaves
¼ cup chopped fresh
  parsley leaves
4 cups cooked wild bay
  shrimp or larger shrimp

1. Make the dressing: In a small bowl, combine the oil, orange zest, orange juice, lemon juice, honey, and salt. Whisk until well incorporated. Set aside.

2. In a medium bowl, combine the orange, tangerine, rice, mint, parsley, and shrimp. Add the dressing and mix the ingredients together. Divide the salad among four individual plates and serve immediately.

3. Store in the refrigerator for up to 2 days.

Ingredient tip: Shrimp is an excellent source of vitamin B_{12} and selenium, which protects from heart disease, type 2 diabetes, and depression. If desired, you can top with slivered or chopped almonds.

Per serving: Calories: 648; Total fat: 28g; Saturated fat: 4g; Cholesterol: 274mg; Sodium: 313mg; Carbohydrates: 60g; Sugar: 12g; Fiber: 2g; Protein: 40g

Crunchy Vegetable & Tuna Salad on Tomatoes

Heart-friendly tuna is rich in omega-3 fatty acids and potassium. We ramp up a typical tuna salad by adding a variety of vegetables and substituting a quick and easy vinaigrette dressing for the traditional mayo.

Serves 4

Prep time: 10 minutes

2 large organic tomatoes

1 teaspoon sea
   salt, divided

Black pepper

3 (5-ounce) cans wild
   albacore tuna in water

½ stalk organic
   celery, chopped

½ English cucumber,
   peeled and chopped

2 scallions, chopped (green
   parts only)

¼ cup chopped
   parsley leaves

½ cup olive oil

2 tablespoons red
   wine vinegar

1 tablespoon freshly
   squeezed lemon juice

1 tablespoon mustard
   or Dijon mustard
   (without garlic)

½ teaspoon sea salt

1. Slice the tomatoes and divide them among four plates. Sprinkle the tomato slices with ½ teaspoon of salt and season them with pepper.

2. Place the tuna in a medium bowl and break it up with a fork. Stir in the celery, cucumber, scallions, and parsley.

3. In a pint jar, combine the oil, vinegar, lemon juice, mustard, and remaining ½ teaspoon salt. Cover and shake vigorously until mixed.

4. Pour the dressing over the tuna salad and mix gently but thoroughly. Scoop one-quarter of the tuna salad over the tomatoes on each plate. Serve immediately.

5. Store in the refrigerator for up to 2 days.

Ingredient tip: Canned tuna is a high-histamine food. Those with histamine intolerance can experience symptoms including rashes, itching, headaches, fatigue, nausea, shortness of breath, or nasal congestion. If you become symptomatic after eating canned foods, speak with a doctor or nutritionist about medicine, supplements, or a low-histamine diet.

Per serving: Calories: 390; Total fat: 30g; Saturated fat: 5g; Cholesterol: 41mg; Sodium: 1296mg; Carbohydrates: 5g; Sugar: 3g; Fiber: 2g; Protein: 24g

Curried Chicken Salad

Chicken salad is so versatile! For this recipe, we went with a delicious mayonnaise-based curry dressing. For variety, you can substitute a cup of halved grapes for the cranberries. Serve this chicken salad by itself, on a bed of lettuce (as tolerated), or in a sandwich or wrap.

Serves 4

Prep time: 15 minutes

½ cup slivered almonds or walnut pieces

½ cup low-FODMAP mayonnaise

¼ cup 24-hour yogurt or low-FODMAP dairy-free yogurt

1 tablespoon freshly squeezed lemon juice

4 teaspoons curry powder

1 teaspoon honey

½ teaspoon sea salt

¼ teaspoon freshly ground black pepper

4 cups cooked chicken, shredded or cut into cubes

2 medium carrots, shredded

1 stalk organic celery, chopped

¼ cup chopped cilantro

¼ cup dried cranberries (optional)

1. In a small saucepan over medium-high heat, cook the almonds for about 5 minutes, stirring frequently, until they are golden brown. Remove the nuts from the pan and set them aside to cool.

2. In a small bowl, whisk together the mayonnaise, yogurt, lemon juice, curry powder, honey, salt, and pepper. Set aside.

3. In a medium bowl, combine the chicken, carrots, celery, cilantro, and cranberries (if using). Spoon the dressing and almonds over the chicken mixture and stir to combine. Serve immediately.

4. Store in the refrigerator for up to 3 days.

SIBO tip: If you want to test your sensitivity to curry, try a very small amount with a different dish that you know you tolerate to see how you do.

Per serving: Calories: 435; Total fat: 31g; Saturated fat: 4g; Cholesterol: 87mg; Sodium: 1081mg; Carbohydrates: 11g; Sugar: 6g; Fiber: 4g; Protein: 28g

BLT Egg Salad

This recipe transforms a basic egg salad into a well-rounded and delicious meal. Enjoy it by itself, over a small salad as in this recipe, with low-FODMAP crackers, or on toast or rice cakes. Save time by precooking bacon at the beginning of the week to use in a variety of dishes.

Serves 4

Prep time: 10 minutes

Cook time: 15 minutes

8 strips bacon, chopped

8 hard-boiled eggs (see The Best Hard-Boiled Eggs, page 31)

⅓ cup low-FODMAP mayonnaise

1 tablespoon mustard (without garlic)

1 teaspoon freshly squeezed lemon juice

¼ teaspoon sea salt

¼ teaspoon freshly ground black pepper

¾ stalk organic celery, finely chopped

2 tablespoons chopped chives

1 pint organic cherry tomatoes, halved

4 large butter lettuce leaves

1. In a large skillet over medium heat, add 1 tablespoon of water and the chopped bacon. Cook for 4 to 6 minutes or until crispy. Set aside.

2. In a medium bowl, mash the eggs into small pieces with a fork. Add the mayonnaise, mustard, lemon juice, salt, and pepper, and mix until incorporated evenly. Add the celery, chives, tomatoes, and cooled bacon and gently mix.

3. Place 1 lettuce leaf each on four plates and top each leaf with a quarter of the egg salad. Serve immediately.

4. Store leftovers in the refrigerator for up to 3 days.

SIBO tip: Some people have an issue digesting the protein in egg whites, while those with fat malabsorption may have an issue with the fat in the yolk. I recommend trying an egg white and an egg yolk at separate times to see if you react to one or the other.

Per serving: Calories: 354; Total fat: 30g; Saturated fat: 7g; Cholesterol: 390mg; Sodium: 710mg; Carbohydrates: 5g; Sugar: 3g; Fiber: 1g; Protein: 18g

Easy Niçoise Salad

This Niçoise salad takes shortcuts by using bagged salad, canned tuna, and pre-boiled eggs. We add a bit of lettuce to this salad for crunch, but aside from the cherry tomatoes, it consists of roasted vegetables and soft ingredients that are easier to digest than those in a traditional salad.

Serves 4

Prep time: 5 minutes

Cook time: 25 minutes

1 pound baby new potatoes, cut into bite-size pieces

½ pound green beans, trimmed

2 tablespoons garlic oil

½ teaspoon sea salt, plus more for sprinkling

¼ teaspoon freshly ground black pepper, plus more for sprinkling

½ cup olive oil

3 tablespoons red wine vinegar

1½ teaspoons mustard

1 bag mixed butter lettuce or baby greens (omit lettuce for (CSD))

1 pint organic cherry tomatoes, halved

INGREDIENT LIST CONTINUES ON NEXT PAGE

1. Preheat the oven to 425°F. Line a baking sheet with a silicone baking mat or parchment paper.

2. Place the potatoes on one end of the baking sheet and the green beans on the other, keeping them separate. Top each with 1 tablespoon garlic oil and sprinkle with salt and pepper. Mix to disperse the oil and seasonings. Cook for 20 minutes, stirring after 10 minutes.

3. Meanwhile, in a pint-size Mason jar, combine the olive oil, vinegar, mustard, ½ teaspoon of salt, and ¼ teaspoon of pepper. Set aside.

4. Divide the lettuce among four plates and top each with cherry tomato halves, sliced egg, tuna, and kalamata olives, leaving space for the potatoes and green beans.

5. Remove the vegetables from the oven and allow them to cool for 5 minutes. Divide them among the plates. Shake the dressing and then drizzle each salad with about 2 tablespoons of dressing. Sprinkle each salad with parsley and serve immediately.

CONTINUED

Easy Niçoise Salad CONTINUED

4 hard-boiled eggs, sliced
(see The Best Hard-Boiled
Eggs, page 31)
3 (5-ounce) cans wild
albacore tuna in water
or olive oil, drained and
broken apart
20 pitted kalamata olives
2 tablespoons
chopped parsley

Speed it up: Use any leftover roasted veggies you may have
in this salad. You can roast a large batch of potatoes over the
weekend to use in so many ways.

Per serving: Calories: 678; Total fat: 48g; Saturated fat: 7g;
Cholesterol: 224mg; Sodium: 1199mg; Carbohydrates: 30g;
Sugar: 5g; Fiber: 5g; Protein: 33g

DAIRY-FREE | EGG-FREE | GLUTEN-FREE | NUT-FREE
DIETS: BPD, CSD, LFD

Thai-Inspired Chicken Noodle Soup

I started this recipe when I was playing around with the classic Thai-inspired soup tom kha gai. I wanted the familiar flavor of that soup, but I also wanted to incorporate more vegetables and rice noodles.

Serves 4
Prep time: 10 minutes
Cook time: 15 minutes

6 cups low-FODMAP
   chicken broth
1 tablespoon grated
   organic lime zest
1 tablespoon grated
   organic lemon zest
2 tablespoons minced
   fresh ginger
1 pound boneless, skinless
   chicken thighs, cut into
   bite-size pieces
1 can coconut milk
2 carrots, peeled and
   thinly sliced
1 bunch bok choy
1 (8-ounce) package thin
   rice noodles
1 tablespoon fish sauce
1 tablespoon freshly
   squeezed lime juice
1 teaspoon sea salt
¼ cup chopped cilantro

1. In a large saucepan or stock pot, combine the chicken broth, lime zest, lemon zest, and ginger and bring the mixture to a boil.

2. Reduce the heat to a simmer, add the chicken, coconut milk, and carrots and simmer for about 5 minutes.

3. Add the bok choy and rice noodles and simmer for about another 3 minutes, until the rice noodles are cooked through. Add the fish sauce, lime juice, and salt. Taste and add more salt as needed.

4. Divide the soup among four bowls and top each with cilantro. Serve immediately or store in the refrigerator for up to 3 days.

SIBO tip: Many people find soup easy to digest and also extremely comforting. It also helps you stay hydrated. If you don't tolerate rice noodles, you can leave them out.

Per serving: Calories: 562; Total fat: 26g; Saturated fat: 15g; Cholesterol: 99mg; Sodium: 2676mg; Carbohydrates: 60g; Sugar: 10g; Fiber: 5g; Protein: 29g

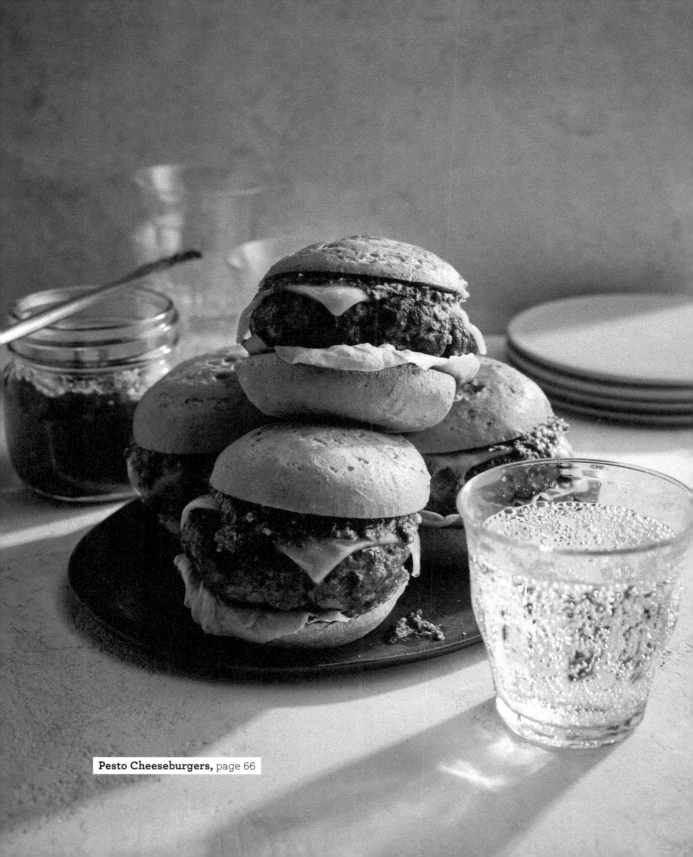

Pesto Cheeseburgers, page 66

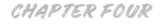

CHAPTER FOUR

Dinner Mains

This chapter highlights easy and delectable main dishes using just one baking sheet to cook the whole meal. Other dishes, like Pesto Cheeseburgers (page 66), give you the option of adding a side dish of your own choice. For a delicious family meal, try the Savory Turkey Meatballs (page 60) and let everyone pick their own sauce, such as Lemony Spinach Pesto (page 102), and decide whether they want their meatballs served over pasta.

Tomato—Bacon Grilled Cheese Sandwich

There are so many possible grilled cheese variations, including ones you could make using some delicious spreads in this book, such as Tapenade (page 99) or Roasted Red Pepper Aioli (page 104). Although bread isn't recommended on all SIBO diets, many people who tolerate rice or potatoes also tolerate white bread.

Serves 4

Prep time: 5 minutes

Cook time: 15 minutes

6 slices bacon

2 large organic
tomatoes, sliced

Sea salt

Freshly ground
black pepper

8 slices low-FODMAP
gluten-free or
sourdough bread

¼ cup butter, melted

¼ pound Gruyère or
cheddar cheese, sliced or
shredded

1. In a large skillet over medium heat, cook the bacon to desired doneness, 3 to 5 minutes per side.

2. Meanwhile, season the tomato slices lightly with salt and pepper and set them aside.

3. Lightly brush one side of each slice of bread with melted butter and set the buttered bread slices aside.

4. Remove the cooked bacon from the pan and drain the bacon grease. In the same pan over medium heat, place 4 slices of bread, buttered side down. Top each with 2 slices of cheese and cover the pan for about 2 minutes, or until the cheese begins to melt and the bread is golden brown. Meanwhile, cut each piece of bacon in half.

5. Uncover the pan. Place 3 pieces of bacon and tomato slices on top of the cheese on each sandwich. Top each sandwich with its second slice of bread, buttered side up. Flip each sandwich over and cook until the second side is golden brown. Serve immediately.

Per serving: Calories: 458; Total fat: 30g; Saturated fat: 15g; Cholesterol: 74mg; Sodium: 789mg; Carbohydrates: 33g; Sugar: 9g; Fiber: 4g; Protein: 17g

EGG-FREE | GLUTEN-FREE

DIETS: BPD, GAPS, LFD, SCD, SSFG

Charcuterie & Cheese Board

Charcuterie boards are not just for appetizers; they also make a really great dinner. They allow us to nibble as we please, use what's available in the fridge, and eat fruits and veggies in a fun way. Put together your own yummy board of deliciousness; the items I've listed here are just suggestions—omit and add on as you like. You can also make this board without gluten, nuts, dairy, or eggs, depending on the ingredients you choose.

Prep time: 10 minutes

Prosciutto (made with just pork and salt)

Low-FODMAP lunch meat, rolled up

Low-FODMAP cheese such as Gruyère, manchego, Brie, cheddar, or goat (choose cheeses aged for 30 days or more for (BPD), (GAPS), (SCD), or (SSFG))

Low-FODMAP crackers (or almond-based crackers for (BPD), (GAPS), (SCD), or (SSFG))

Warm Citrus & Garlic Olives (page 85)

Raw or roasted nuts or seeds (almonds, Brazil nuts, hazelnuts, macadamia nuts, peanuts, pecans, pumpkin seeds, or walnuts)

Dried cranberries

Low-FODMAP sourdough or gluten-free bread, cut into cubes (omit for (BPD), (GAPS), (SCD), or (SSFG))

Artichoke & Pesto Dip (page 86)

Zesty Cilantro Sauce (page 103)

Fresh fruit such as grapes or berries

Fresh vegetables such as peeled and sliced cucumber, carrots, bell pepper, or zucchini

Canned artichoke hearts

Hard-boiled eggs with Tapenade (page 99) or Low-FODMAP hot sauce

Mint sprigs

On a large cutting board, arrange the ingredients artfully so that colors, shapes, and textures contrast. For items with liquid, arrange them in small bowls on the cutting board. Enjoy!

Nutritional Information depends on specific ingredients and amounts. Check the low-FODMAP app listed in Resources (page 108) for low-FODMAP amounts.

Coconut Lemon Scallops

Scallops can be a bit of a splurge. However, if you love scallops, making this dish at home is much more cost-effective than eating it at a restaurant, and you won't have to guess or inquire about the ingredients. Make sure to ask for dry scallops at the seafood counter. Those that aren't dry are treated with a solution that makes it difficult to get a good sear on the scallop.

Serves 4

Prep time: 10 minutes

Cook time: 20 minutes

2 scallions, sliced (green parts only)

2 tablespoons white vinegar

1 cup canned coconut milk

Grated zest of 1 organic lemon (approximately 2 teaspoons)

Grated zest of 1 organic lime (approximately 1 teaspoon)

2 thin slices ginger

2 teaspoons freshly squeezed lime juice

½ teaspoon fish sauce

1. In a small saucepan over low heat, combine the scallions and vinegar and simmer until the vinegar reduces almost entirely, 2 to 3 minutes.

2. Add the coconut milk, lemon zest, lime zest, and ginger, increase the heat to medium-high, and bring to a simmer. Reduce the heat to medium-low and simmer for 5 minutes. Remove from the heat, add the lime juice and fish sauce, stir, and set aside.

3. Rinse and pat dry the scallops. Season them with the salt and pepper. Melt the coconut oil in a large skillet over medium heat. When the oil is shimmering but not smoking, add the scallops and sear on each side for 2 to 3 minutes or until cooked through. Set aside.

4. Strain the sauce through a fine sieve. In each of four wide bowls, place 1 cup of cooked white rice (if using). Place the scallops on top of the rice and pour the sauce over the top. Sprinkle the bowls with the cilantro and serve immediately. This dish is best served fresh.

1¼ pounds large dry
   scallops
½ teaspoon sea salt
¼ teaspoon freshly ground
   black pepper
1 tablespoon coconut oil
4 cups cooked white rice
   (optional) (omit for ,
   SCD, or SSFG)
2 tablespoons chopped
   cilantro

SIBO tip: Many people with SIBO are sensitive to spicy food. But if you're one of the lucky people who can do chile peppers, hot sauce, or other spicy items, feel free to add them to this or any other dish. Just be aware of any symptoms that may arise.

Per serving: Calories: 445; Total fat: 15g; Saturated fat: 12g; Cholesterol: 36mg; Sodium: 946mg; Carbohydrates: 53g; Sugar: 3g; Fiber: 1g; Protein: 23g

GLUTEN-FREE | NUT-FREE

DIETS: BPD, GAPS, LFD, SCD, SSFG

Quick Lemon & Herb Cod

Cod is a mild white fish that is rich in omega-3 fatty acids and has been shown to improve mood and decrease depression. This dish is best immediately after cooking, so I suggest you only make the amount you will be eating. This recipe is very easy to halve: Just use half of all the ingredients—no other changes are needed.

Serves 4

Prep time: 5 minutes

Cook time: 10 minutes

1 teaspoon sea salt

½ teaspoon freshly ground
   black pepper

1 teaspoon
   smoked paprika

4 cod fillets (1¼ to
   1½ pounds each)

4 tablespoons butter or
   ghee, divided

½ lemon, cut into
   four wedges

1 tablespoon parsley
   leaves, chopped

1. In a small bowl, mix together the salt, pepper, and paprika. Dry the cod fillets and sprinkle each, on both sides, with the spice mixture.

2. In a large skillet over medium heat, melt 2 tablespoons of butter. Add the cod pieces. Cook for 2 minutes and then flip the cod, top with the remaining 2 tablespoons of butter, and cook for another 3 to 4 minutes or until cooked through.

3. Transfer the cod to individual plates, squeeze a lemon wedge over each fillet, and sprinkle each with parsley. Serve immediately.

Ingredient swaps: This is a very simple preparation, and some slight changes will make it feel like a new recipe. Try leaving out the paprika and parsley and topping instead with the Zesty Cilantro Sauce (page 103) or Great Green Sauce (page 98) at the very end.

Per serving: Calories: 213; Total fat: 12g; Saturated fat: 8g; Cholesterol: 104mg; Sodium: 806mg; Carbohydrates: 1g; Sugar: <1g; Fiber: <1g; Protein: 25g

Easy Salmon Cakes

Salmon is an excellent source of vitamins D and B_{12}—two vitamins commonly deficient among people with SIBO. A recent study found that salmon contains bioactive peptides that help control inflammation in the digestive tract and support joint cartilage.

Serves 4
Prep time: 5 minutes
Cook time: 25 minutes

2 tablespoons extra-virgin olive oil, divided, plus more if needed

3 scallions, finely sliced (green parts only)

1 small red bell pepper, finely minced

2 large eggs

3 (6-ounce) cans canned wild salmon, drained

1 tablespoon garlic oil

½ cup almond flour

¼ cup plus
⅓ cup low-FODMAP mayonnaise, divided

1 tablespoon low-FODMAP Dijon mustard

⅓ cup finely chopped fresh parsley

4 tablespoons finely chopped fresh dill, divided

INGREDIENT LIST
CONTINUES ON NEXT PAGE

1. In a large skillet over medium heat, heat 1 tablespoon of olive oil. Add the scallions and bell pepper and sauté for about 5 minutes, until soft. Remove from the heat and set aside.

2. In a large bowl, beat the eggs. Add the salmon, garlic oil, almond flour, ¼ cup of mayonnaise, mustard, parsley, 2 tablespoons of dill, salt, pepper, and cooled scallions and bell pepper. Mix well and form into patties, using 2 to 3 tablespoons of the mixture for each patty.

3. In the same skillet over medium heat, heat the remaining tablespoon of olive oil. Working in batches if needed, cook the patties for 3 to 4 minutes per side. Add another tablespoon of oil as needed.

4. In a small bowl, whisk together the lemon zest, lemon juice, remaining ⅓ cup of mayonnaise, yogurt, and remaining 2 tablespoons of dill. Taste and add salt and pepper as desired.

5. Divide the salmon cakes among four plates and spoon some sauce over them. Serve immediately or refrigerate for up to 2 days.

CONTINUED

1 teaspoon sea salt

½ teaspoon freshly ground
black pepper

Grated zest of 1 organic
lemon (approximately
2 teaspoons)

2 tablespoons freshly
squeezed lemon juice

⅓ cup 24-hour yogurt
or low-FODMAP
dairy-free yogurt

Ingredient swaps: If you want to use fresh salmon, swap
the canned salmon for a pound of cooked salmon, and omit
¼ cup of the mayonnaise. Feel free to use another sauce,
such as the Green Goddess Dressing (page 38), Great Green
Sauce (page 98), or Roasted Red Pepper Aioli (page 104).

Per serving: Calories: 618; Total fat: 51g; Saturated fat: 8g;
Cholesterol: 184mg; Sodium: 1430mg; Carbohydrates: 7g;
Sugar: 3g; Fiber: 3g; Protein: 33g

Parchment-Baked Salmon & Potatoes

If you haven't used parchment for cooking fish, try it! It makes cleanup quick and results in delicious fish. There are many online videos that demonstrate how to wrap fish in parchment paper, so take a minute or two to watch one if you haven't tried it before.

Serves 4

Prep time: 5 minutes

Cook time: 20 minutes

¼ cup garlic oil

1 tablespoon freshly squeezed lemon juice

1 tablespoon chopped fresh dill

1 teaspoon sea salt

½ teaspoon freshly ground black pepper

2 small russet potatoes, peeled and thinly sliced (omit for (GAPS), (SCD), or (SSFG))

4 salmon fillets (4 to 6 ounces each)

1 lemon, thinly sliced

4 tablespoons Green Goddess Dressing (page 38) (optional)

1. Preheat the oven to 400°F. Tear off four large pieces of parchment paper, fold each piece in half, and set the folded paper aside.

2. In a small bowl, mix together the garlic oil, lemon juice, dill, salt, and pepper.

3. Place a quarter of the potatoes in the middle of one half of a piece of parchment paper, slightly overlapping. Place one salmon fillet over the potatoes. Drizzle the salmon with a quarter of the oil mixture and top with a quarter of the lemon slices. Repeat with the other 3 fillets.

4. Fold over the edges of the parchment paper for each piece of salmon to make half-moon shapes. Place the packets on a baking sheet. Cook for 18 to 20 minutes or until cooked through.

5. Unwrap the salmon and remove it from the parchment. Place each piece with its potatoes on a plate. Top each fillet with 1 tablespoon of the Green Goddess Dressing (if using) and serve immediately.

Per serving: Calories: 322; Total fat: 18g; Saturated fat: 3g; Cholesterol: 55mg; Sodium: 760mg; Carbohydrates: 17g; Sugar: 3g; Fiber: 2g; Protein: 24g

DAIRY-FREE | GLUTEN-FREE
DIETS: BPD, CSD, GAPS, LFD, SCD, SSFG

Savory Turkey Meatballs

Meatballs are easy to double or triple and freeze for later. Going to a party? Defrost some cocktail-size meatballs and serve them with a low-FODMAP barbecue sauce or Lemony Spinach Pesto (page 102). Need a quick lunch? Pop some meatballs on a sandwich with Tomato Sauce (page 105) or Zesty Cilantro Sauce (page 103), or use them as your protein in a warm bowl with vegetables and rice.

Serves 4

Prep time: 5 minutes

Cook time: 25 minutes

⅓ cup plus 1 tablespoon almond flour

2 tablespoons low-FODMAP chicken broth

4 scallions, finely chopped (green parts only)

2 teaspoons garlic oil

½ pound ground turkey

½ pound ground pork

1 large egg

1 tablespoon Italian seasoning

1 teaspoon sea salt

½ teaspoon freshly ground black pepper

½ cup organic spinach, finely chopped (optional)

low-FODMAP barbecue sauce (optional)

1. Preheat the oven to 425°F. Line a baking sheet with aluminum foil and place a large wire baking rack over the foil.

2. In a large bowl, combine the almond flour, broth, scallions, oil, turkey, pork, egg, Italian seasoning, salt, pepper, and spinach (if using). Mix with your clean hands until all is well combined.

3. Divide the mixture into 12 equal portions and roll them into balls. Place the meatballs on the wire rack and bake for 20 to 25 minutes or until cooked through.

4. Serve the meatballs immediately with the barbecue sauce or another sauce of your choice. Store in the refrigerator for up to 3 days or freezer for up to 3 months.

Ingredient swaps: If you prefer turkey to pork or the opposite, you can use one pound of either instead of using a half pound of each. If you use ground turkey, try to go with ground dark meat—it has more fat and delivers more flavor.

Per serving: Calories: 372; Total fat: 27g; Saturated fat: 8g; Cholesterol: 132mg; Sodium: 691mg; Carbohydrates: 4g; Sugar: 1g; Fiber: 2g; Protein: 22g

Chicken Piccata

Enjoy this restaurant specialty in just 30 minutes! If possible, choose pasture-raised organic chicken. Labeling requirements for chicken allow marketers to say things like "cage-free" or "pastured" without the chickens getting much actual time outdoors, so if you can, find out where your meat comes from and how it is raised.

Serves 4

Prep time: 5 minutes

Cook time: 25 minutes

4 boneless, skinless
   chicken breasts (1 to
   1½ pounds each)

Sea salt

Freshly ground
   black pepper

⅔ cup white rice flour

1 tablespoon garlic oil

2 tablespoons ghee

½ cup dry white wine
   (optional)

¼ cup freshly squeezed
   lemon juice

¼ cup low-FODMAP
   chicken broth (use ⅓ cup
   if not using wine)

3 tablespoons butter, sliced

3 tablespoons
   capers, drained

1 tablespoon chopped
   fresh parsley

1. Place the chicken breasts between two pieces of plastic wrap and pound them to ½-inch thickness. Dry the breasts with a paper towel and season both sides with salt and pepper.

2. Place the flour in a shallow pan and dredge the chicken in the flour, shaking off any excess. Set aside.

3. In a large skillet over medium-high heat, warm the garlic oil and ghee. Cook the chicken for 3 to 4 minutes per side, until cooked through, working in batches as needed. Set aside the cooked chicken.

4. Pour the wine (if using) into the skillet and cook for about 2 minutes or until reduced by half. If not using wine, skip to the next step.

5. Add the lemon juice, broth, butter, and capers to the skillet, stirring for about 2 minutes. Return the chicken to the pan for 2 minutes. Plate the chicken and sauce and sprinkle with parsley. Serve immediately.

Make it easier: If you don't own a meat mallet, you can use a rolling pin, an empty wine bottle, or a large heavy skillet to pound and flatten chicken breasts. Many online videos detail this simple process.

Per serving: Calories: 394; Total fat: 22g; Saturated fat: 11g; Cholesterol: 120mg; Sodium: 347mg; Carbohydrates: 22g; Sugar: 1g; Fiber: 1g; Protein: 27g

Balsamic-Mustard Chicken with Kale & Tomatoes

Kale is an excellent source of many vitamins and minerals. It also contains the most lutein compared to more than 5,000 other foods. Lutein plays a key role in eye health. Kale is also supportive of the body's detoxification system.

Serves 4

Prep time: 10 minutes

Cook time: 20 minutes

3 tablespoons balsamic vinegar (with no added sugar)

3 tablespoons garlic oil, divided

1 tablespoon honey

1 tablespoon low-FODMAP Dijon mustard

1¼ pounds boneless, skinless chicken thighs, cut into 1-inch strips

½ teaspoon sea salt, divided

¼ teaspoon freshly ground black pepper, divided

1 bunch kale, spines removed and roughly chopped

1 pint organic cherry tomatoes, halved

1. In a small bowl, whisk together the vinegar, 1 tablespoon of oil, honey, and mustard. Set aside.

2. Dry the chicken strips with paper towels, and season both sides with ¼ teaspoon of salt and ⅛ teaspoon of pepper.

3. In a large skillet over medium-high heat, heat the remaining 2 tablespoons of oil. Add the chicken and sear until golden brown, about 3 minutes on each side. Remove the chicken from the pan and set aside.

4. Reduce the heat to medium. In the same pan, combine the kale and tomatoes and season them with the remaining ¼ teaspoon of salt and ⅛ teaspoon of pepper. Cook for about 3 minutes, stirring occasionally, or until the greens are wilted and the tomatoes are soft.

5. Return the chicken to the pan along with the vinegar mixture. Mix together and cook for about 7 more minutes, until the sauce thickens and the chicken is cooked through. Serve immediately, over rice if desired. Store in the refrigerator for up to 3 days.

Per serving: Calories: 303; Total fat: 20g; Saturated fat: 2g; Cholesterol: 114mg; Sodium: 600mg; Carbohydrates: 10g; Sugar: 8g; Fiber: 2g; Protein: 24g

EGG-FREE | GLUTEN-FREE | NUT-FREE
DIETS: BPD, GAPS, LFD, SCD, SSFG

Cheesy Veggie-Stuffed Chicken

Thick chicken breasts work great in this recipe because you'll have enough room to stuff in veggies. Since chicken breasts don't contain as much fat as chicken thighs, it's important to not overcook them so they'll stay tender and tasty. The chicken is cooked when the thickest part reaches 160°F.

Serves 4

Prep time: 10 minutes

Cook time: 20 minutes

4 boneless, skinless
   chicken breasts
½ teaspoon sea salt
¼ teaspoon freshly ground
   black pepper
1 small zucchini, peeled,
   halved lengthwise, and
   thinly sliced
1 small red bell pepper,
   thinly sliced
1 small organic
   tomato, chopped
½ cup chopped green or
   black olives
1 tablespoon garlic oil
2 teaspoons Italian
   seasoning (without garlic)
1 cup shredded mozzarella
   or other cheese (choose
   cheeses aged for 30 days
   or more for BPD, GAPS,
   SCD, or SSFG)
1 scallion, sliced
   (green parts only)

1. Preheat the oven to 425°F. Line a baking sheet with parchment paper or aluminum foil.

2. Sprinkle the chicken breasts on both sides with the salt and pepper and place them on the lined baking sheet.

3. Using a knife, make multiple vertical slits close together and most of the way through each chicken breast. Stuff each slit with the zucchini and bell pepper. Stuff the tomatoes and olives in between the slits. Drizzle the stuffed breasts with the garlic oil and sprinkle them with the Italian seasoning, cheese, and scallions.

4. Bake for about 20 minutes or until the chicken is cooked through. Serve immediately or refrigerate for up to 3 days.

Speed it up: To save time, use low-FODMAP salsa in place of the fresh tomatoes. Or if you have Tomato Sauce (page 105) on hand, you can spread a tablespoon or two over the vegetables and then top it with the cheese.

Per serving: Calories: 286; Total fat: 16g; Saturated fat: 6g; Cholesterol: 95mg; Sodium: 621mg; Carbohydrates: 5g; Sugar: 2g; Fiber: 2g; Protein: 32g

Balsamic-Glazed Pork Chops

Bone-in pork chops make for tastier, juicier chops that won't dry out during the cooking process, thanks to the collagen in the bones. The fat that surrounds the bones flavors the surrounding meat. Fat helps keeps us satiated in between meals, supports healthy hair and skin, and helps us absorb fat-soluble vitamins.

Serves 4

Prep time: 5 minutes

Cook time: 15 minutes

4 bone-in pork chops

¾ teaspoon sea salt, divided

½ teaspoon plus ⅛ teaspoon freshly ground black pepper, divided

2 tablespoons avocado oil

¼ cup balsamic vinegar (with no added sugar for (SCD), (GAPS), (SSFG), or (BPD))

¼ cup maple syrup (use for (LFD)) or honey (use for (BPD), (GAPS), (SCD), or (SSFG))

1 tablespoon garlic oil

1 tablespoon chopped fresh rosemary

¼ cup butter, cubed

1. Dry the pork chops with a paper towel. Sprinkle both sides of the chops with ½ teaspoon of salt and ½ teaspoon of pepper.

2. In a large skillet over medium-high heat, heat the avocado oil. Add the pork chops and cook for 5 to 7 minutes on each side, or to an internal temperature of 160°F for medium. Remove the chops from the pan and set them aside.

3. Reduce the heat to medium-low. In the same pan, whisk together the vinegar, sweetener, garlic oil, rosemary, the remaining ¼ teaspoon of salt, and the remaining ⅛ teaspoon of pepper. Simmer for 3 to 5 minutes, stirring intermittently. Remove the pan from the heat and whisk in the butter until it is melted.

4. Place a pork chop on each plate and top each chop with the sauce. Serve immediately.

Speed it up: Instead of fresh rosemary, try using 1 teaspoon of dried rosemary or 1 teaspoon of Italian seasoning.

Per serving: Calories: 469; Total fat: 34g; Saturated fat: 11g; Cholesterol: 96mg; Sodium: 599mg; Carbohydrates: 16g; Sugar: 14g; Fiber: <1g; Protein: 23g

Rosemary-Orange Pork Tenderloin with Potatoes

This flavorful pork tenderloin takes minimal preparation, and adding the potatoes to the same baking sheet saves time and cleanup. I recommend purple potatoes because they contain more antioxidants than white potatoes.

Serves 4
Prep time: 5 minutes
Cook time: 25 minutes

3 tablespoons
    low-FODMAP
    Dijon mustard
1 tablespoon honey
1 tablespoon maple syrup
2 tablespoons freshly
    squeezed orange juice
Grated zest of
    1 organic orange
2 teaspoons
    finely chopped
    rosemary, divided
1¼ pounds organic
    potatoes, cut into
    bite-size pieces
2 tablespoons extra-virgin
    olive oil
1 (1¼-pound) pork
    tenderloin, dried with a
    paper towel
1 teaspoon sea salt
½ teaspoon black pepper

1. Preheat the oven to 425°F. Line a baking sheet with aluminum foil and set it aside.

2. In a small bowl, combine the mustard, honey, maple syrup, orange juice, orange zest, and 1 teaspoon of rosemary. Whisk to incorporate and set the mustard sauce aside.

3. In the middle of the lined baking sheet, combine the remaining 1 teaspoon of rosemary with the potatoes and oil. Toss everything together until the potatoes are evenly coated. Move the potatoes to the sides of the pan.

4. Place the tenderloin in the middle of the baking sheet. Sprinkle the potatoes and tenderloin with salt and pepper. Drizzle the mustard sauce over the tenderloin and the potatoes.

5. Bake for 20 to 25 minutes, or until the internal temperature reaches 145°F for medium-rare or 160°F for medium. Remove the pan from the oven. Let the meat rest while you serve the potatoes, and then cut the meat against the grain and serve it immediately.

Per serving: Calories: 356; Total fat: 11g; Saturated fat: 2g; Cholesterol: 92mg; Sodium: 930mg; Carbohydrates: 30g; Sugar: 14g; Fiber: 4g; Protein: 33g

Pesto Cheeseburgers

Burgers invite all kinds of variations, such as different sauces, condiments, or toppings like bacon, a slice of avocado, or, in this case, pesto. If you don't care for pesto, you can still use this burger as your go-to recipe; just omit the pesto and adjust the salt and pepper as desired.

Serves 4

Prep time: 5 minutes

Cook time: 20 minutes

1 pound ground beef

⅓ pound ground pork

⅔ cup Lemony Spinach
   Pesto, divided (page 102)

Sea salt

Freshly ground
   black pepper

4 slices cheddar or
   Gruyère cheese

4 low-FODMAP burger
   buns (omit for (BPD),
   (GAPS), (SCD), or (SSFG)) or 8 large
   butter lettuce leaves
   (optional)

1. In a large bowl, mix the beef, pork, and ⅓ cup of pesto. Form the meat mixture into 4 large patties. Sprinkle the patties with salt and pepper.

2. Heat a large skillet over medium heat. Add the burgers and cook for 7 minutes on one side. Flip the burgers and place a slice of cheese on top of each burger. Cook for 5 more minutes.

3. Meanwhile, spread 2 teaspoons of pesto on each of the buns or leaves (if using). Place the hot burgers on the buns or leaves or plate the burgers, and top each burger with 2 teaspoons of pesto. Serve immediately.

Make it easier: Double or triple this recipe and freeze the extra burgers or use them for lunches or dinners throughout the week. Burgers are a great family dinner. Let everyone choose their favorite toppings, type of bun, and side dish, and everyone will be happy.

Per serving: Calories: 787; Total fat: 52g; Saturated fat: 16g; Cholesterol: 153mg; Sodium: 745mg; Carbohydrates: 33g; Sugar: 5g; Fiber: 2g; Protein: 47g

One-Sheet Beef & Broccoli

You don't have go out to eat to have food that reminds you of your favorite Chinese restaurant. The sauce in this dish is fairly salty, so you don't need to add salt to the meat or vegetables. If you don't tolerate starch, leave out the tapioca starch and water and just let the sauce reduce while the beef and broccoli cook.

Serves 4

Prep time: 5 minutes

Cook time: 10 minutes

½ cup coconut aminos

2 tablespoons garlic oil

2 tablespoons sesame oil

2 tablespoons rice vinegar

2 tablespoons peeled chopped fresh ginger

1 tablespoon honey

1 tablespoon whole cane sugar (optional)

3 to 4 cups broccoli florets (depending on your tolerance)

1¼ pounds flank steak, sliced against the grain into bite-size pieces

1 teaspoon tapioca starch or arrowroot starch (optional)

½ cup cold water (optional)

4 cups cooked white rice, warm

2 scallions, sliced (green parts only), for garnish

1. Preheat the oven to 425°F. Line a baking sheet with parchment paper or aluminum foil and set it aside.

2. In a large bowl, combine the coconut aminos, garlic oil, sesame oil, vinegar, ginger, honey, and sugar (if using), and whisk to incorporate. Add the broccoli to the mixture and stir to coat.

3. Spread the steak in a single layer on the lined baking sheet. Using tongs, remove the broccoli from the marinade and place it on the baking sheet with the steak, spreading the florets in a single layer around the steak. Bake the steak and broccoli for about 12 minutes or until cooked through.

4. Meanwhile, transfer the marinade into a small saucepan and bring it to a boil over medium-high heat. In a small bowl, whisk the tapioca starch and cold water together (if using); then stir the mixture into the marinade to thicken it. Reduce the heat to low. (If not using the starch, keep the marinade over medium heat until the steak is ready. It will reduce slightly.)

5. Place 1 cup of cooked rice each in four wide bowls or plates. Top with the beef and broccoli mixture. Top each dish with a quarter of the sauce and garnish with the scallions (if using). Serve immediately or refrigerate for up to 3 days.

Per serving: Calories: 614; Total fat: 24g; Saturated fat: 6g; Cholesterol: 92mg; Sodium: 635mg; Carbohydrates: 59g; Sugar: 11g; Fiber: 2g; Protein: 36g

"Sloppy Joes" over Baked Potato Halves

In this version of sloppy joes, I use a baked potato instead of the typical bun. If you tolerate bread, you can certainly eat it that way, too. We also sneak some veggies into this version, and since they're grated and finely chopped, picky eaters are unlikely to notice them. If you don't tolerate spinach or carrots, go ahead and remove them.

Serves 4

Prep time: 10 minutes

Cook time: 20 minutes

2 medium organic potatoes or small sweet potatoes

3 tablespoons water, divided

1 tablespoon avocado or olive oil

4 scallions, chopped (green parts only)

1 large carrot, grated

1 pound ground beef or ground turkey

1 tablespoon organic tomato paste

1 cup low-FODMAP organic ketchup

2 tablespoons low-FODMAP mustard (without garlic)

1 tablespoon honey

1. Scrub and dry the potatoes. Poke each potato with a knife in four different places. Place the potatoes on a microwave-safe plate, pour 1 tablespoon of water onto the plate, and microwave on high for 5 minutes. Flip the potatoes. Push a steak knife into the middle of each potato. If there is a lot of give, the potato is done. Otherwise, microwave for another 3 to 5 minutes.

2. Meanwhile, in a large skillet over medium heat, heat the oil. Add the scallions and sauté for about 3 minutes until they are beginning to soften. Add the carrots and cook for 1 minute. Add the ground beef, breaking it up and stirring intermittently until no pink remains, about 8 minutes.

3. Add the tomato paste, ketchup, mustard, honey, vinegar, remaining 2 tablespoons of water, spinach, liquid smoke (if using), and hot sauce (if using) to the skillet and stir to combine. Bring the mixture to a low simmer and cook for about 8 minutes. Add a little more water if needed for consistency.

1 tablespoon apple
cider vinegar

1 cup spinach,
finely chopped

¼ teaspoon liquid smoke
(optional)

Dash low-FODMAP hot
sauce (optional)

1 teaspoon sea salt

Freshly ground
black pepper

4. Meanwhile, cut the potatoes in half, place one potato half on each plate, and break up the insides of the potato halves with a fork. When the meat is done, scoop a quarter of the mixture over each potato. Serve immediately or refrigerate for up to 3 days.

Make it easier: This is a great recipe to double or triple and freeze for a quick defrosted meal. These sloppy joes are also great to reheat for lunch in the microwave.

Per serving: Calories: 498; Total fat: 22g; Saturated fat: 8g; Cholesterol: 100mg; Sodium: 1317mg; Carbohydrates: 43g; Sugar: 20g; Fiber: 4g; Protein: 32g

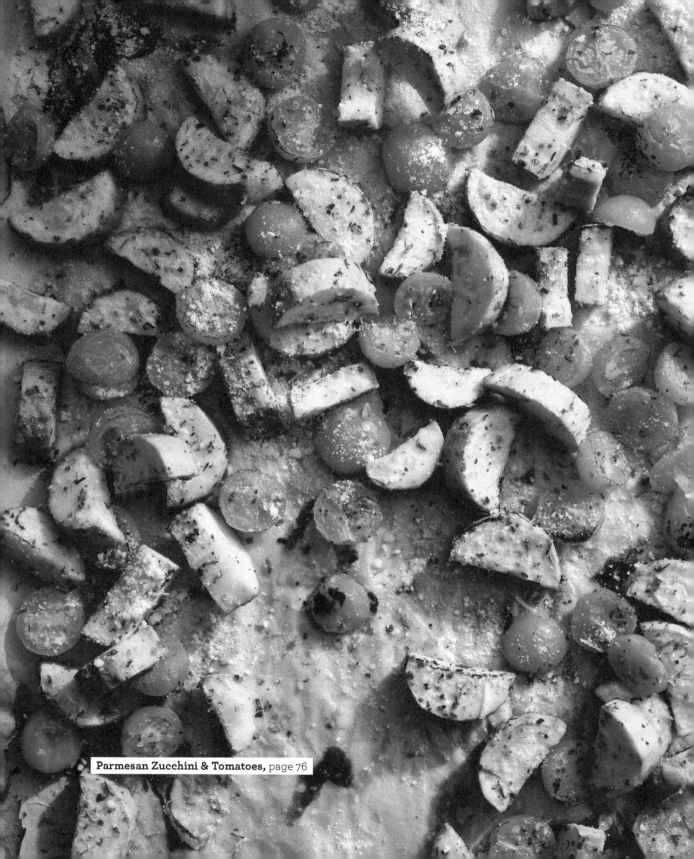

Parmesan Zucchini & Tomatoes, page 76

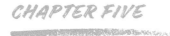
Simple Sides

The following side dishes are big on taste. Pair one of these sides with a main dish or put a couple of side dishes together for a light vegetarian supper. The Maple & Five-Spice Roasted Sweet Potatoes (page 77) go great with Parchment-Baked Salmon & Potatoes (page 59), and they would go equally great with Creamy Herb-Scrambled Eggs (page 32) if you like "breakfast for dinner" as much as I do. If you're just starting on a SIBO diet, try the Garlic Mashed Potatoes (page 79), Broccoli Potato Soup (page 81), or Pureed Carrots with Coriander & Lime (page 74), as pureed foods are easier to digest.

Fruit Salad with Honey-Yogurt Dressing

It's recommended to start a SIBO diet with peeled, seeded, and cooked vegetables and fruit. This salad is raw, so if you're unsure of your tolerance, start with a very small serving. You can also replace any of the fruits in this recipe with fruits that you tolerate. Just double-check the low-FODMAP amounts for any fruits you add.

Serves 4 to 6

Prep time: 15 minutes

½ cup 24-hour yogurt
 or low-FODMAP
 non-dairy yogurt
1 tablespoon plus
 1 teaspoon honey
1 teaspoon vanilla extract
1 cup organic strawberries,
 quartered
1 cup organic
 grapes, halved
1 cup blueberries
2 kiwifruit, peeled
 and sliced
2 tangerines, peeled and
 sectioned
1 large banana, sliced

In a large bowl, whisk the yogurt, honey, and vanilla until blended. Add the strawberries, grapes, blueberries, kiwifruit, tangerines, and banana, and stir to coat the fruit. Serve immediately. This salad is best fresh but can be stored in the refrigerator for up to 2 days.

Speed it up: Buying prewashed and precut fruits and berries is a time-saving option.

Per serving: Calories: 176; Total fat: 2g; Saturated fat: 1g; Cholesterol: 3mg; Sodium: 12mg; Carbohydrates: 41g; Sugar: 30g; Fiber: 5g; Protein: 3g

DAIRY-FREE | EGG-FREE | GLUTEN-FREE | NUT-FREE | VEGETARIAN
DIETS: BPD, CSD, GAPS, LFD, SCD, SSFG

Roasted Rosemary Carrots

In addition to being tolerated well by many people with SIBO, carrots are versatile and can be pureed, steamed, roasted, or used in soups. Since you want as much variety in your vegetable choices as possible, try mixing your carrots with other vegetables that aren't recommended in higher amounts, such as Brussels sprouts.

Serves 4
Prep time: 5 minutes
Cook time: 20 minutes

6 or 7 medium carrots
1 tablespoon chopped
  fresh rosemary
2 tablespoons olive oil
1 teaspoon sea salt
½ teaspoon freshly ground
  black pepper

1. Preheat the oven to 400°F. Line a baking sheet with aluminum foil and set it aside.

2. Peel the carrots and slice them thinly on the bias. For the widest part of the carrot, cut each piece in half so they're about the same size as the other pieces.

3. Place the carrots, rosemary, oil, salt, and pepper on the lined baking sheet. Toss the ingredients to mix them all and to evenly coat the carrots.

4. Cook for 10 minutes. Stir and cook for 7 to 10 more minutes. Remove the carrots from the oven and serve them immediately or store them in the refrigerator for up to 5 days.

Speed it up: Baby carrots make preparation time easier and quicker, as they don't need to be peeled or sliced. You can also substitute a teaspoon of dried herbs or a favorite spice for the rosemary or forgo herbs or spices altogether.

Per serving: Calories: 99; Total fat: 7g; Saturated fat: 1g; Cholesterol: 0mg; Sodium: 648mg; Carbohydrates: 9g; Sugar: 4g; Fiber: 3g; Protein: 1g

Pureed Carrots with Coriander & Lime

FODMAPs are not detected in carrots, so you don't have to worry about sticking to a particular portion size. Try this side with Cheesy Veggie-Stuffed Chicken (page 63), Quick Lemon & Herb Cod (page 56), or Parchment-Baked Salmon & Potatoes (page 59).

Serves 4

Prep time: 5 minutes

Cook time: 15 minutes

1 pound whole
   baby carrots

2 tablespoons olive oil,
   coconut oil, or ghee

1 teaspoon ground
   coriander

Juice and grated zest of
   1 organic lime

½ teaspoon sea salt

¼ teaspoon freshly ground
   black pepper

1. Place the carrots in a medium saucepan, cover them with water, and bring to a boil over high heat. Reduce the heat to medium and simmer for 8 to 10 minutes, or until the carrots are very soft.

2. Meanwhile, in a food processor, combine the oil, coriander, lime zest, lime juice, salt, and pepper. Drain the carrots and add them to the food processor. Process until the carrots are fully pureed and all ingredients are incorporated. Serve immediately or store in the refrigerator for up to 5 days.

Ingredient swaps: If you're just starting a diet, try this puree with just the carrots, oil, and salt. As you expand your diet, try the carrot puree with sweet or savory ingredients. For instance, to make the carrots sweet for breakfast or dessert, you can add cinnamon and honey. For savory options, trade out other spices or top them with chopped fresh herbs.

Per serving: Calories: 103; Total fat: 7g; Saturated fat: 1g; Cholesterol: 0mg; Sodium: 382mg; Carbohydrates: 11g; Sugar: 6g; Fiber: 3g; Protein: 1g

Grilled Eggplant

Grilled eggplant is delicious hot or chilled and is also great on sandwiches. Because of the eggplant skin's health benefits, we don't peel it, but if you are just starting a diet and are highly symptomatic, you can peel the skin and it won't change the recipe.

Serves 4

Prep time: 5 minutes

Cook time: 25 minutes

1 large eggplant

2 teaspoons sea
  salt, divided

¼ cup garlic oil

¼ cup extra-virgin olive oil

¼ cup balsamic vinegar
  (optional)

½ teaspoon freshly ground
  black pepper

1. Cut the eggplant into ¼-inch-thick rounds and set the rounds on paper towels. Sprinkle the rounds on both sides with 1 teaspoon of salt and let them sit for 10 minutes.

2. Meanwhile, in a large bowl, combine the garlic oil, olive oil, balsamic vinegar (if using), the remaining 1 teaspoon of salt, and the pepper, and mix together.

3. Use a paper towel to wipe off each eggplant round, removing the salt and excess moisture. Place a large grill pan or large skillet over medium-high heat. Brush each eggplant slice with the oil mixture on both sides.

4. Working in batches if needed, cook the eggplant for about 5 minutes on the first side, turn over, and cook for another 2 minutes. Brush each slice with any remaining oil mixture and serve immediately. Store any leftovers in the refrigerator for up to 4 days.

Make it easier: If you own an outdoor grill, this is the perfect recipe for grilling.

Per serving: Calories: 283; Total fat: 27g; Saturated fat: 4g; Cholesterol: 0mg; Sodium: 296mg; Carbohydrates: 10g; Sugar: 6g; Fiber: 5g; Protein: 2g

Parmesan Zucchini & Tomatoes

Some people are nervous about eating nightshade vegetables like tomatoes because it's widely assumed that they cause inflammation. However, there isn't any scientific study supporting that claim. People with SIBO have a variety of intolerances, and if tomatoes are one of yours, then just leave them out for 3 or 4 weeks before testing them again in a tasty dish like this one.

Serves 6
Prep time: 10 minutes
Cook time: 10 minutes

2 medium zucchini, peeled and sliced into half rounds (about 2 cups)

1 pint organic cherry tomatoes, halved

1 teaspoon Italian seasoning

½ teaspoon sea salt

¼ freshly ground black pepper

½ cup grated Parmesan cheese, divided

1. Preheat the oven to 425°F. Line a baking sheet with a silicone baking mat, aluminum foil, or parchment paper.

2. Place the zucchini, cherry tomatoes, Italian seasoning, salt, pepper, and ¼ cup Parmesan cheese on the lined baking sheet. Mix everything together well and spread the mixture evenly. Sprinkle the remaining ¼ cup of Parmesan cheese over the mixture.

3. Bake for 7 minutes; then turn the oven to broil. Broil the zucchini and tomatoes for 3 to 4 minutes and remove them from the oven. This dish is best served immediately, but it can be stored in the refrigerator for up to 4 days.

SIBO tip: Normally, we recommend peeling and seeding vegetables, but of course that would be very labor intensive with cherry tomatoes! Since the tomatoes are cooked, they'll be easier to digest. Just chew well, making sure each bite is liquid in your mouth before you swallow.

Per serving: Calories: 55; Total fat: 3g; Saturated fat: 1g; Cholesterol: 7mg; Sodium: 158mg; Carbohydrates: 5g; Sugar: 3g; Fiber: 1g; Protein: 4g

Maple & Five-Spice Roasted Sweet Potatoes

Chinese five-spice powder can be used in both sweet and savory dishes. It's a combination of fennel, cinnamon, star anise, Szechuan pepper, and cloves, said to encompass the five flavors of sweet, sour, bitter, salty, and umami. You can buy five-spice powder in most grocery stores or make it yourself by combining the five spices. If you don't like the flavor of Chinese five-spice powder, try a teaspoon of cinnamon in this recipe instead.

Serves 5

Prep time: 5 minutes

Cook time: 20 minutes

1 medium orange-fleshed
    sweet potato

2 tablespoons olive oil

1 tablespoon maple syrup

½ teaspoon sea salt

1 teaspoon Chinese
    five-spice powder

1. Preheat the oven to 425°F. Line a baking sheet with parchment paper or a silicone baking mat.

2. Peel the sweet potato and cut it into small, bite-size cubes. Place them on the lined baking sheet along with the oil, syrup, salt, and five-spice powder. Toss to fully coat the potatoes.

3. Bake for 10 minutes, stir, and bake for another 5 to 7 minutes or until slightly crispy and tender. Serve immediately or keep refrigerated for up to 5 days.

SIBO tip: When someone first starts a SIBO diet, I recommend they start with potatoes as a starchy vegetable. If they tolerate potatoes, I then recommend sweet potatoes. They are low-FODMAP in ½-cup portions.

Per serving: Calories: 80; Total fat: 5g; Saturated fat: 1g; Cholesterol: 0mg; Sodium: 251mg; Carbohydrates: 8g; Sugar: 4g; Fiber: 1g; Protein: <1g

Parsnip Fries

If you've never tried a parsnip, maybe it's time! Parsnips look like white carrots because they are part of the carrot family. A great source of vitamin C, parsnips also contain 2.8 grams of fiber per ½ cooked cup. Normally this would be great, but for those with SIBO, sometimes higher amounts of fiber may cause symptoms. If you know you tolerate fiber well, parsnips will probably work for you. If you're not sure, start with a small serving.

Serves 4
Prep time: 10 minutes
Cook time: 20 minutes

1¼ pounds parsnips, peeled and cut into French fry strips
1 tablespoon olive oil
1 teaspoon sea salt
¼ teaspoon freshly ground black pepper
1 tablespoon white truffle oil (optional)
½ cup grated Parmesan cheese (optional)

1. Preheat the oven to 400°F. Line a baking sheet with a silicone baking mat or parchment paper.

2. Place the parsnips on the lined sheet and cover them with the olive oil, salt, and pepper. Toss well and spread over the baking sheet evenly.

3. Bake for 10 minutes. Flip the fries and bake them for 10 more minutes. Remove the fries from the oven, top them with the truffle oil and Parmesan cheese (if using), and toss together. Serve immediately.

Ingredient swaps: We use parsnips in this recipe to add variety, but if you tolerate potatoes, they work well in this recipe, too.

Per serving: Calories: 137; Total fat: 4g; Saturated fat: 1g; Cholesterol: 0mg; Sodium: 599mg; Carbohydrates: 26g; Sugar: 7g; Fiber: 7g; Protein: 2g

Garlic Mashed Potatoes

I recommend organic potatoes in this recipe because potatoes are among the conventionally raised produce with the highest pesticide residue. So even if your budget doesn't allow for buying organic across the board, consider buying organic for fruits and vegetables that are listed in the Dirty Dozen (see page 108). If you prefer a stronger garlic flavor, you can add 1 more tablespoon of garlic oil and use 1 less tablespoon of butter.

Serves 4 to 6
Prep time: 5 minutes
Cook time: 25 minutes

2 pounds organic Yukon Gold potatoes, peeled and halved

2 tablespoons garlic oil

6 tablespoons butter, softened

⅔ cup warm low-FODMAP chicken broth or warm low-FODMAP milk of choice

1 teaspoon sea salt

½ teaspoon freshly ground black pepper

1. Place the potatoes in a large pot and cover them with warm water approximately 2 inches over the potatoes. Bring to a boil over high heat. Reduce the heat to medium-high and cook for about 20 minutes, or until the potatoes are fork-tender.

2. Drain the potatoes and place them in a medium bowl. Add the garlic oil, butter, broth, salt, and pepper. Using the whisk attachment on a hand mixer, whip the potatoes until they are soft and uniform with no visible chunks.

3. Serve immediately or store in the refrigerator for up to a week.

SIBO tip: I often recommend peeled white potatoes for those starting a SIBO diet. White potatoes are high-glycemic, so for those who tolerate starch, they are easy to digest and don't cause symptoms. They are helpful for those who enjoy carbs and feel deprived without them. They are also critical for those who are underweight or experiencing unwanted weight loss.

Per serving: Calories: 399; Total fat: 24g; Saturated fat: 12g; Cholesterol: 47mg; Sodium: 889mg; Carbohydrates: 42g; Sugar: 5g; Fiber: 3g; Protein: 5g

DAIRY-FREE | EGG-FREE | GLUTEN-FREE | VEGETARIAN

DIETS: BPD, CSD, LFD

Creamy Coconut Rice

Coconut milk adds extra healthy fat to help keep you satiated so you're less likely to snack in-between meals. If you use a different type of rice, make sure to check the package instructions for the recommended amount of liquid and cooking time.

Serves 4

Prep time: 5 minutes

Cook time: 25 minutes

1 cup white jasmine rice

1 cup coconut milk

⅔ cup water

4 teaspoons unsweetened shredded coconut (optional)

Grated zest of 1 organic lime

1 teaspoon freshly squeezed lime juice

1. Rinse and drain the rice.

2. In a medium saucepan, combine the rice, coconut milk, and water. Bring to a boil and then reduce the heat to a simmer. Cover and simmer for 15 minutes. Remove from the heat and leave covered for 9 minutes.

3. Meanwhile, in a small sauté pan, stir the coconut (if using) over medium-low heat until it is lightly golden brown, 3 to 5 minutes. Remove the coconut from the heat and set aside.

4. Fluff the rice; then stir in the lime zest and lime juice. Divide the rice into four bowls and top each bowl of rice with the toasted shredded coconut. Serve immediately or store in the refrigerator for up to 5 days.

SIBO tip: Coconut milk is low-FODMAP at ¼ cup. However, not everyone tolerates coconut products. For those who do, coconut milk adds healthy fat and delicious taste to recipes. This is a good basic recipe to try if you know that you tolerate white rice.

Per serving: Calories: 263; Total fat: 11g; Saturated fat: 9g; Cholesterol: 0mg; Sodium: 6mg; Carbohydrates: 39g; Sugar: 2g; Fiber: 2g; Protein: 4g

DAIRY-FREE | EGG-FREE | GLUTEN-FREE | NUT-FREE | VEGETARIAN
DIETS: BPD, CSD, LFD

Broccoli Potato Soup

This comforting soup makes a great side dish or quick lunch. Broccoli, part of the cruciferous vegetable family, is not something everyone does well with right away. Trying broccoli in a soup like this where it's partially or fully pureed will make it easier to digest. If you do tolerate broccoli, it has many health benefits, its anti-inflammatory and antioxidant properties being two of its strongest.

Serves 4

Prep time: 10 minutes

Cook time: 20 minutes

2 tablespoons avocado or olive oil

4 scallions, sliced (green parts only)

2 cups chopped broccoli

2 small russet potatoes, peeled and cut into bite-size cubes

3½ cups low-FODMAP chicken or vegetable broth

1 teaspoon freshly squeezed lemon juice

1 teaspoon sea salt

¼ teaspoon ground mustard

¼ teaspoon freshly ground black pepper

1. Heat a medium Dutch oven or soup pot over medium-high heat. Pour the oil into the pot and then add the scallions. Sauté for 2 minutes. Reduce the heat to medium, add the broccoli and potatoes, and sauté for 3 more minutes.

2. Pour the broth over the vegetables, increase the heat to high, and bring to a boil. Reduce the heat to medium and cook until the vegetables are tender, about 15 minutes.

3. Using a handheld blender, puree the soup in the pot. Alternatively, carefully puree the soup in a blender in two batches. Add the lemon juice, salt, mustard, and pepper, and adjust the seasoning to taste. Serve immediately or store in the refrigerator for up to 4 days.

Speed it up: I recommend buying bagged precut broccoli heads. They are available at Trader Joe's and other stores. You can use them in this soup as well as to make roasted or steamed broccoli for a quick and easy side.

Per serving: Calories: 158; Total fat: 7g; Saturated fat: 1g; Cholesterol: 4mg; Sodium: 1406mg; Carbohydrates: 19g; Sugar: 3g; Fiber: 2g; Protein: 4g

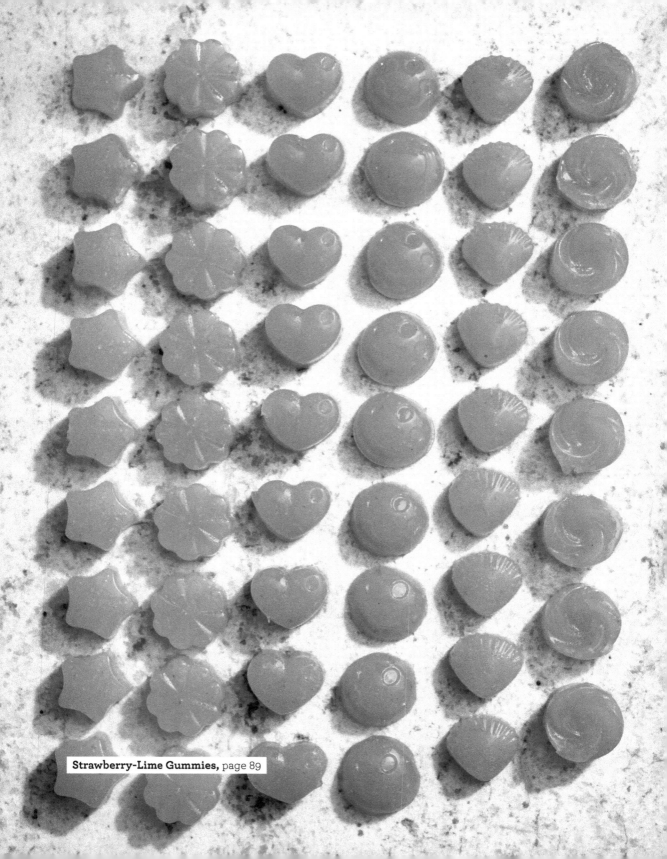

Strawberry-Lime Gummies, page 89

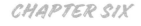

CHAPTER SIX

Sweet Treats & Snacks

Sometimes you need a snack when you're on the run. Try the Cinnamon-Cumin Nuts (page 84) or Maple-Pecan Nut Butter (page 87). If you're looking for the perfect appetizer to take to a party so you can have something safe to snack on, you'll want to make the Warm Citrus & Garlic Olives (page 85) or Artichoke & Pesto Dip (page 86). Or maybe you just want a quick and easy dessert after dinner to quiet a sweet tooth. The Caramelized Pineapple (page 91) or Warm Honey–Balsamic Strawberries (page 90) will do the trick for you and the whole family.

Cinnamon-Cumin Nuts

These mixed nuts make a lovely hostess or holiday gift, and they're highly portable. Nuts are delicious by themselves, or they can be chopped and used to top yogurt or salads. Nuts can be hard to digest, so make sure to keep your consumption within amounts that you tolerate.

Serves 6

Prep time: 5 minutes

Cook time: 20 minutes

1⅓ cups almonds

1⅓ cup hazelnuts

1⅓ cup walnuts

3 tablespoons maple syrup

2 tablespoons coconut oil
   or olive oil

2 teaspoons cinnamon

2 teaspoons sea salt (plus
   more as desired)

1 teaspoon cumin

1. Preheat the oven to 350°F. Line a baking sheet with parchment paper, aluminum foil, or a silicone baking mat.

2. On the baking sheet, place the almonds, hazelnuts, walnuts, maple syrup, coconut oil, cinnamon, salt, and cumin. Mix thoroughly, and spread the nuts evenly over the pan.

3. Bake for 10 minutes. Stir and bake for another 5 to 10 minutes until fragrant. Remove from the oven, stir, and let cool for 5 minutes. Taste and add more salt as desired.

Ingredient swaps: Switch out any low-FODMAP nuts or seeds (like pumpkin seeds) in this recipe—just use 3 cups of nuts and/or seeds overall. You can also use different spice or herb combinations.

Per serving: Calories: 544; Total fat: 50g; Saturated fat: 7g; Cholesterol: 0mg; Sodium: 873mg; Carbohydrates: 20g; Sugar: 9g; Fiber: 7g; Protein: 13g

DAIRY-FREE │ EGG-FREE │ GLUTEN-FREE │ NUT-FREE │ VEGETARIAN
DIETS: CSD, LFD

Warm Citrus & Garlic Olives

These olives taste great right after heating, but the flavor will continue to improve over time, so make a double batch! Everything but the olives is meant only for flavoring, so, for example, don't eat the garlic cloves. They will give a nice garlic flavor to the oil, but they are still high-FODMAP and shouldn't be consumed.

Serves 4

Prep time: 5 minutes

Cook time: 10 minutes

1 (12-ounce) jar green
    olives, whole

Peel of 1 organic tangerine
    or small organic orange

¼ cup extra-virgin olive oil

2 garlic cloves, cut in
    3 slices each

2 thyme sprigs

1 teaspoon fennel seeds

1. Drain the olives and place them in a small saucepan. Add the citrus peel, oil, garlic, thyme sprigs, and fennel seeds.

2. Over medium-low heat, warm the olives for about 7 minutes or until they are heated through and the mixture is fragrant. Transfer to a serving dish and serve immediately or store in the refrigerator for up to 5 days.

Ingredient swaps: Try different herb combinations in this olive dish, such as rosemary, tarragon, or basil. You can also use different citrus, such as lime or lemon. If you don't like the taste of garlic, you can certainly leave that out.

Per serving: Calories: 186; Total fat: 20g; Saturated fat: 3g; Cholesterol: 0mg; Sodium: 699mg; Carbohydrates: 2g; Sugar: 0g; Fiber: 2g; Protein: 1g

Artichoke & Pesto Dip

This hearty dip can be paired with crackers or veggies for a delicious appetizer at home or to take to a potluck or party. Many people don't know that canned artichoke hearts are low-FODMAP (in ½-cup servings) because the FODMAPs leach into the canning water.

Serves 6

Prep time: 5 minutes

Cook time: 15 minutes

1 can artichoke hearts, drained and chopped

½ cup low-FODMAP mayonnaise (without garlic)

½ cup Lemony Spinach Pesto (page 102)

½ cup grated Parmesan cheese

¼ teaspoon sea salt

1. Preheat the oven to 400°F.

2. In a small bowl, mix together the artichoke hearts, mayonnaise, pesto, Parmesan cheese, and salt. Spoon the mixture into a 1¼-quart casserole dish, spreading it evenly.

3. Bake for 15 minutes. Remove the dip from the oven and serve it immediately with low-FODMAP crackers or vegetables or store it in the refrigerator for up to 3 days. Reheat the dip in the microwave or oven.

Speed it up: Instead of baking the dip, you can microwave it on medium-high for 2 minutes, stir, and then microwave for another 3 minutes. Stir again and serve immediately.

Per serving: Calories: 251; Total fat: 23g; Saturated fat: 4g; Cholesterol: 15mg; Sodium: 641mg; Carbohydrates: 6g; Sugar: 1g; Fiber: 1g; Protein: 4g

DAIRY-FREE | EGG-FREE | GLUTEN-FREE | VEGETARIAN

DIETS: BPD, CSD, GAPS, LFD, SCD, SSFG

Maple-Pecan Nut Butter

Since nuts are hard to digest, I typically recommend that people first try nut milk. If you tolerate nut milk, then try nut butter. A teaspoon of nut butter can help stave off a sweet tooth or serve as a welcome addition to yogurt, low-FODMAP toast, or a banana.

Makes about 2 cups

Prep time: 10 minutes

Cook time: 10 minutes

1 pound raw pecans

2 tablespoons maple syrup or honey (optional) (use honey for (BPD), (GAPS), (SCD), or (SSFG))

1 teaspoon sea salt

1. Preheat the oven to 350°F.

2. Spread the raw pecans evenly on a baking sheet. Bake for 11 minutes. Remove from the oven and cool for 10 minutes.

3. Place the pecans in a food processor and blend for about 3 minutes, or until the pecans turn into butter, stopping to scrape down the sides if necessary. Once the pecans are a thick liquid, add the maple syrup (if using) and salt. Blend for 30 more seconds. Serve immediately or store in the refrigerator for up to 3 weeks.

Ingredient swaps: Add a variety of spices, seeds, or other ingredients as desired. If you tolerate seeds, you can add chia seeds. Try flavor combinations like vanilla extract with cinnamon or cardamom. Add coconut oil to the butter and/or coconut flakes if you like extra texture. For a savory nut butter, try adding curry or cayenne pepper.

Per serving (1 tablespoon): Calories: 100; Total fat: 10g; Saturated fat: 1g; Cholesterol: 0mg; Sodium: 73mg; Carbohydrates: 2g; Sugar: 1g; Fiber: 1g; Protein: 1g

Bacon Banana Rice Cakes

This quick and easy snack or light lunch combines sweet and savory for something that seems childlike but is equally satisfying for adults. If you don't tolerate or enjoy rice cakes, you can also use low-FODMAP gluten-free or sourdough toast or Sweet Potato Toast (page 33).

Serves 4

Prep time: 5 minutes

Cook time: 10 minutes

2 slices bacon, chopped

¼ cup Maple-Pecan Nut Butter (page 87) or nut butter of your choice

4 rice cakes

2 small bananas, sliced (use unripe for (LFD))

4 teaspoons honey

1. Heat a medium skillet over medium heat. Place the bacon in the hot pan and cook until crisp, about 7 minutes. Transfer the bacon to a paper towel to drain. Set aside.

2. Spread 1 tablespoon of nut butter on each rice cake. Place the banana slices on top of the nut butter. Drizzle 1 teaspoon of honey over each rice cake and top each with bacon pieces. Serve immediately.

Make it easier: Make extra bacon over the weekend for an on-the-go breakfast or snack throughout the week.

Per serving: Calories: 216; Total fat: 10g; Saturated fat: 2g; Cholesterol: 4mg; Sodium: 152mg; Carbohydrates: 28g; Sugar: 14g; Fiber: 3g; Protein: 6g

Strawberry-Lime Gummies

These gummies are a fun and healthy treat, and making them is a great family activity. I have a ton of different molds for various holidays, so gummies are often served for special occasions at my house. I love that they keep well, and gelatin, as tolerated, is very healing for the gut. Make sure to buy a quality brand made from grass-fed cows for the greatest benefit. (See Resources on page 108 for recommended brands.)

Serves 6
Makes approximately 25 gummies, depending on mold size
Prep time: 5 minutes, plus 15 minutes to chill
Cook time: 10 minutes

½ cup fresh lime juice
3 tablespoons gelatin
½ cup organic strawberries (from fresh or defrosted strawberries)
⅓ cup clover honey
½ teaspoon vanilla extract

1. Place the lime juice in a small saucepan and sprinkle the gelatin over it. Meanwhile, puree the strawberries in a blender or using a hand blender.

2. Add the strawberries and honey to the saucepan. Heat and whisk as everything melts, 3 to 5 minutes. Remove the pan from the heat and add the vanilla.

3. Pour the mixture into candy molds or an 8-inch-by-8-inch glass pan. Let set in the refrigerator for 15 minutes or until solid. Remove the gummies from the molds or cut them into squares. Store the gummies in the refrigerator for up to a week.

Ingredient swaps: You can try a variety of different flavors of gummies, using fruit purees or juice, low-FODMAP milk, and even melted chocolate. Just make sure that you end up with one cup of liquid for the gummies—in this recipe it's the ½ cup lime juice and ½ cup strawberry puree.

Per serving: Calories: 88; Total fat: <1g; Saturated fat: 0g; Cholesterol: 0mg; Sodium: 7mg; Carbohydrates: 18g; Sugar: 16g; Fiber: <1g; Protein: 6g

DAIRY-FREE | EGG-FREE | GLUTEN-FREE | NUT-FREE | VEGETARIAN
DIETS: BPD, CSD, GAPS, LFD, SCD, SSFG

Warm Honey–Balsamic Strawberries

Fresh strawberries don't need anything when they're at their best, but in this recipe, we bring in a sophisticated balsamic-vinegar-and-honey combination to bring them to the next level. Balsamic strawberries are delicious by themselves for dessert or chilled atop 24-hour yogurt. Buy the best-quality aged balsamic vinegar that you can afford; quality makes a difference.

Serves 4

Prep time: 5 minutes

Cook time: 5 minutes

1 tablespoon balsamic vinegar (without added sugar for 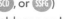 BPD, GAPS, SCD, or SSFG)

1 tablespoon honey

2 cups organic strawberries, quartered

1 teaspoon vanilla extract

In a medium sauté pan over medium-high heat, combine the vinegar and honey. Stir as the honey melts. Add the strawberries and sauté for 2 minutes. Remove the pan from the heat and stir in the vanilla. Serve immediately.

Ingredient swaps: Try a little melted chocolate on top of the sautéed strawberries or add some orange rind during the sauté process. You can even use other flavored vinegars that you may have on hand. Try out whatever sounds good—that's the fun part of cooking!

Per serving: Calories: 47; Total fat: <1g; Saturated fat: 0g; Cholesterol: 0mg; Sodium: 2mg; Carbohydrates: 11g; Sugar: 9g; Fiber: 2g; Protein: 1g

DAIRY-FREE | EGG-FREE | GLUTEN-FREE | NUT-FREE | VEGETARIAN
DIETS: BPD, CSD, GAPS, LFD, SCD, SSFG

Caramelized Pineapple

This recipe with just three ingredients creates a quick yet delectable dessert. When you're choosing a pineapple, start by smelling the bottom of the fruit. It should have a light but distinctive pineapple smell. Additionally, it should look fresh, have green leaves and a greenish-yellow exterior, and feel firm but have a slight give to it.

Serves 4

Prep time: 5 minutes

Cook time: 10 minutes

2 tablespoons butter or coconut oil

1 tablespoon plus 1 teaspoon honey

4 cups fresh pineapple chunks

In a sauté pan over medium heat, melt the butter. Add the honey and stir to combine. Add the pineapple chunks and sauté for 3 to 4 minutes or until heated through. Serve immediately or store in the refrigerator for up to 3 days, and reheat before serving.

Ingredient swaps: Try adding a sprinkle of cinnamon during the cooking process or topping the pineapple with toasted coconut. You can also drizzle it with a bit of melted chocolate if you're feeling especially decadent.

Per serving: Calories: 155; Total fat: 6g; Saturated fat: 4g; Cholesterol: 15mg; Sodium: 48mg; Carbohydrates: 28g; Sugar: 22g; Fiber: 2g; Protein: 1g

No-Bake Chocolate Nut Butter Balls

To me, these nut butter balls taste a bit like the chocolate chip cookie dough we're not supposed to eat before we bake it! But this treat is healthy to eat raw. We add coconut oil for some healthy fat and collagen for its gut-healing properties. Nevertheless, make sure to be judicious with serving amounts. This recipe incorporates nut butter and nut flour, so you won't want to overdo it.

Makes 12 balls

Prep time: 15 minutes

½ cup Maple-Pecan Nut
   Butter (page 87) or nut
   butter of your choice
⅓ cup almond flour
¼ cup honey
2 tablespoons collagen
   (optional)
1 tablespoon coconut oil
1 teaspoon vanilla extract
⅓ cup non-dairy mini
   or regular-size dark
   chocolate chips

1. In a bowl, combine the nut butter, flour, honey, collagen (if using), coconut oil, and vanilla and mix well. Add the chocolate chips and mix again. Place the mixture in the freezer for 10 minutes to firm up.

2. Roll the mixture into 12 balls. Enjoy the balls immediately or store them in the refrigerator for up to a week.

Make it easier: Double or triple this recipe and freeze the balls for up to 3 months. Take them out a couple at a time for snacks on the go, or bring a bigger batch with you to work or a party. One thing I know about being on a SIBO diet is that it's always important to have food in the freezer!

Per serving: Calories: 141; Total fat: 10g; Saturated fat: 3g; Cholesterol: 0mg; Sodium: 46mg; Carbohydrates: 12g; Sugar: 7g; Fiber: 3g; Protein: 4g

DAIRY-FREE | EGG-FREE | GLUTEN-FREE | NUT-FREE | VEGETARIAN
DIETS: CSD, LFD

Rich Hot Chocolate

Make this hot chocolate in advance and then refrigerate it for yummy cold chocolate milk or reheat it when you're ready for a warm beverage. Mix the hot chocolate with some espresso for a delightful morning mocha.

Serves 4

Prep time: 5 minutes

Cook time: 5 minutes

4 cups low-FODMAP milk
of choice

2 tablespoons maple syrup

2 heaping tablespoons
plus 2 heaping teaspoons
cocoa powder

2 teaspoons vanilla extract

1. In a medium saucepan over medium heat, heat the milk and maple syrup for about 5 minutes, stirring to incorporate.

2. When the milk is warm, add the cocoa powder and whisk to incorporate. Remove the pan from the heat and add the vanilla. Serve immediately. Hot chocolate may be stored in the refrigerator for up to 5 days.

Speed it up: To make hot chocolate in the microwave, divide the maple syrup and cocoa among four mugs. Add a table-spoon of milk to each mug and mix it with the maple syrup and cocoa. Divide the rest of the milk among the mugs and stir. Microwave each mug on high for 1 minute or until hot. Stir ½ teaspoon of vanilla extract into each mug and serve.

Per serving: Calories: 76; Total fat: 3g; Saturated fat: <1g; Cholesterol: 0mg; Sodium: 173mg; Carbohydrates: 10g; Sugar: 6g; Fiber: 1g; Protein: 2g

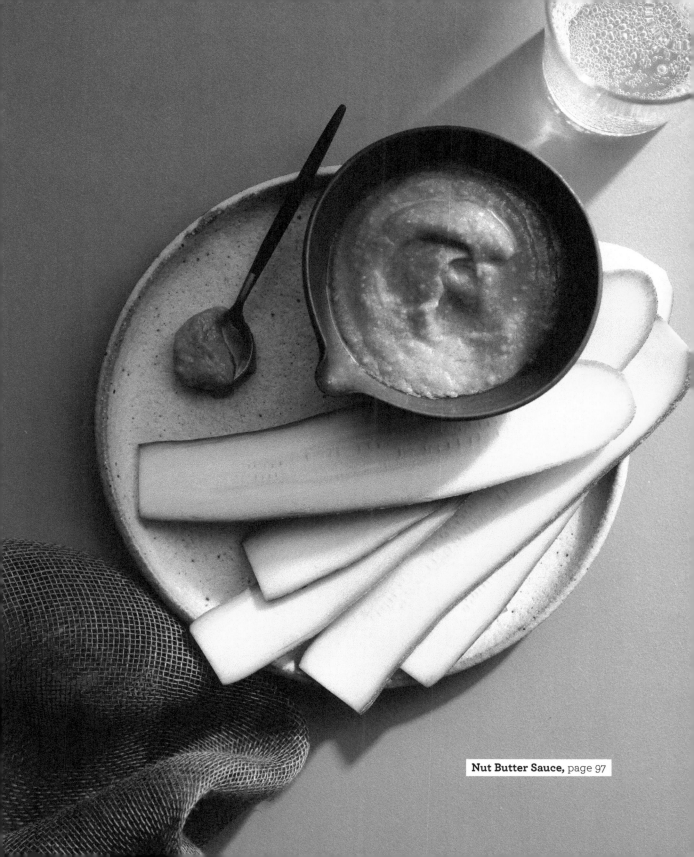

Nut Butter Sauce, page 97

CHAPTER SEVEN

Basic Staples, Condiments, Dressings & More

This chapter may seem basic, but these recipes are lifesavers. Sauces, condiments, and dressings such as Nut Butter Sauce (page 97) or Great Green Sauce (page 98) can change roasted vegetables or a piece of meat into a completely different meal. Homemade Rice Milk (page 96) or Simple Syrup (page 101) allows you to create your own healthy and inexpensive drinks at home. Tapenade (page 99), Zesty Cilantro Sauce (page 103), and Roasted Red Pepper Aioli (page 104) all make great dips for low-FODMAP crackers or vegetables.

Homemade Rice Milk

Making your own rice milk at home is very simple and can save you money, especially if you purchase large amounts of rice at once. You can also freeze rice milk for up to a month. Rice milk can be used in any recipe that calls for low-FODMAP milk. It's low-FODMAP in ¾-cup servings.

Makes 4½ cups

Prep time: 5 minutes

4 cups water

1 cup cooked white rice

1 tablespoon honey or
  maple syrup (optional)

1. In a blender, combine the water, cooked rice, and sweetener (if using). Blend for 1 minute and then let it settle. Blend again for 1 minute. Taste and add more sweetener if desired.

2. Serve immediately or store in the refrigerator for up to 5 days.

Ingredient swaps: Rice milk is great on its own as a base, but you can also create many different milk flavors. Add soft fruit such as strawberries when you blend the rice milk for a delicious fruity milk, or sprinkle in cinnamon and vanilla extract.

Per serving (¾ cup): Calories: 34; Total fat: <1g; Saturated fat: 0g; Cholesterol: 0mg; Sodium: <1mg; Carbohydrates: 7g; Sugar: 0g; Fiber: <1g; Protein: 1g

Nut Butter Sauce

This quick and easy nut butter sauce is delicious over meats, vegetables, low-FODMAP pasta, vegetable noodles, or rice. It's also wonderful as a dip for low-FODMAP crackers or vegetables. Really, most food items are just a vehicle for this delectable sauce! If you don't have coconut aminos, soy sauce is low-FODMAP in the amount used in this recipe and can be substituted. Read your labels if you are avoiding gluten, though, as many soy sauces do contain gluten.

Makes 1 cup
Prep time: 5 minutes

⅓ cup plus 1 tablespoon
    rice vinegar
⅓ cup plus 1 tablespoon
    almond butter or other
    nut butter of choice
¼ cup olive oil or
    avocado oil
2 tablespoons
    coconut aminos
2 tablespoons minced
    peeled fresh ginger

In a medium bowl, combine the vinegar, almond butter, olive oil, coconut aminos, and minced ginger. Whisk together until well mixed. Serve immediately or store in the refrigerator for up to 5 days.

Speed it up: Look for online videos on how to peel ginger with a spoon. Yes, a spoon! Though I adore the taste and depth of fresh ginger in a recipe, you can always substitute 2 teaspoons of powdered ginger in this recipe.

Per serving (1 tablespoon): Calories: 71; Total fat: 7g; Saturated fat: 1g; Cholesterol: 0mg; Sodium: 48; Carbohydrates: 2g; Sugar: 1g; Fiber: 1g; Protein: 1g

DAIRY-FREE | EGG-FREE | GLUTEN-FREE | VEGETARIAN
DIETS: BPD, CSD, GAPS, LFD, SCD, SSFG

Great Green Sauce

A little avocado makes this sauce creamy and smooth. Use this sauce as a spread or dressing, or drizzle it over meat or veggie bowls. Serve some with your next Charcuterie & Cheese Board (page 53). Many people miss avocado on a SIBO diet since it is only low-FODMAP in serving sizes of ⅛ an avocado. However, I've had clients who tolerate it in larger amounts because it only contains one FODMAP—sorbitol. You can test a moderate-high-FODMAP amount, a quarter of an avocado, to see whether it creates symptoms.

Makes about 2 cups
Prep time: 5 minutes

1 small or medium avocado
½ cup parsley leaves
½ cup cilantro leaves
Juice and grated zest of
    1 organic lemon
½ cup water
¼ cup olive oil
¼ cup garlic oil
½ teaspoon sea salt
½ cup walnut pieces

1. In a food processor, combine the avocado, parsley, cilantro, lemon zest, lemon juice, water, olive oil, garlic oil, salt, and walnuts. Process until smooth, about 1 minute, stopping to scrape down the sides as needed.

2. Serve immediately or store in the refrigerator for up to a week.

Ingredient swaps: Substitute any combination of herbs you like, such as cilantro, parsley, mint, chives, basil, chervil, or tarragon—just make sure you end up with 1 cup of herbs.

Per serving (2 tablespoons): Calories: 99; Total fat: 11g; Saturated fat: 1g; Cholesterol: 0mg; Sodium: 75mg; Carbohydrates: 2g; Sugar: <1g; Fiber: 1g; Protein: 1g

Tapenade

Tapenade goes with so many things! It's delicious as a dip for crackers or vegetables, on top of grilled meats or vegetables, and with some recipes in this book, such as Parmesan Zucchini & Tomatoes (page 76). Because the kalamata olives and capers are already quite salty, there's no need to add any salt to this recipe. You can add fresh herbs to this recipe instead of dried herbs, but using dried herbs makes it come together much quicker.

Makes 1 cup

Prep time: 5 minutes

1 (12-ounce) jar kalamata olives, drained

2 tablespoons capers

2 tablespoons garlic oil

2 teaspoons freshly squeezed lemon juice

1 teaspoon anchovy paste

½ teaspoon Italian seasoning (without garlic)

1. In a food processor, combine the olives, capers, oil, lemon juice, anchovy paste, and Italian seasoning. Process until slightly chunky but well incorporated, stopping to scrape down the sides as needed.

2. Spoon the tapenade into a small bowl and serve it immediately or store it in the refrigerator for up to 5 days.

SIBO tip: I often recommend olives as part of a healthy meal. Because olives contain healthy fat, they can help you stay satiated between meals. It's recommended to leave 4 to 5 hours in between any caloric intake in order to support the sweeping wave of the small intestine, the migrating motor complex (MMC).

Per serving (2 tablespoons): Calories: 135; Total fat: 13g; Saturated fat: 1g; Cholesterol: <1mg; Sodium: 691mg; Carbohydrates: 5g; Sugar: 0g; Fiber: <1g; Protein: <1g

DAIRY-FREE | EGG-FREE | GLUTEN-FREE | NUT-FREE | VEGETARIAN
DIETS: BPD, CSD, GAPS, LFD, SCD, SSFG

Cinnamon-Orange Cranberry Sauce

Enjoy cranberry sauce year-round on sandwiches, ham, turkey, or roast beef—not just over the holidays! I love the tartness balanced by the sweetness. I've made many different cranberry sauce recipes over the years, and this one is definitely a favorite with its hints of orange and cinnamon.

Makes about 1½ cups
Prep time: 5 minutes
Cook time: 25 minutes

10 ounces fresh or frozen
cranberries
Grated zest of
1 organic orange
½ cup freshly squeezed
orange juice or water (use
water for (BPD))
⅓ cup maple syrup or
honey (use maple syrup
for (LFD); use honey for
(BPD), (GAPS), (SCD), or (SSFG))
½ teaspoon cinnamon

1. In a medium saucepan over medium-high heat, combine the cranberries, orange zest, orange juice, sweetener, and cinnamon. Mix the ingredients and bring them to a boil. Reduce the heat and simmer, stirring occasionally, for about 20 minutes or until the sauce thickens and most of the berries have popped.

2. Serve immediately or store in the refrigerator for up to a week.

Ingredient swaps: Try different spices or other ingredients in this recipe to make it your own. In addition to cinnamon, try nutmeg or allspice, or simply replace the ½ teaspoon of cinnamon with ½ teaspoon of Chinese five-spice powder. You can also add chopped nuts, such as pecans.

Per serving (2 tablespoons): Calories: 23; Total fat: 0g; Saturated fat: 0g; Cholesterol: 0mg; Sodium: 1mg; Carbohydrates: 6g; Sugar: 4g; Fiber: 1g; Protein: <1g

Simple Syrup

Simple syrup is something that you may have heard of being used in cocktails, but it's also great to have on hand to make your own lemonade or limeade or to add to iced tea or coffee or other cold drinks that benefit from a sweetener. If you like, you can add herbs like basil or spices like cardamom to create a flavored syrup.

Makes 1⅓ cups

Cook time: 20 minutes

1 cup honey or sugar (use honey for BPD, GAPS, SCD, or SSFG; use sugar for LFD)

1 cup water

1. In a small saucepan over medium heat, combine the sweetener and water. Stir occasionally for 7 to 8 minutes or until the sweetener is dissolved and fully mixed with the water.

2. Remove the syrup from the heat, let it cool for 10 minutes, and either use it immediately or store it in the refrigerator for up to 1 month.

Speed it up: Place the honey or sugar and water in a microwave-safe container and microwave on high for 3 minutes. Stir and cool for 10 minutes.

Per serving (2 tablespoons): Calories: 98; Total fat: 0g; Saturated fat: 0g; Cholesterol: 0mg; Sodium: 1mg; Carbohydrates: 27g; Sugar: 27g; Fiber: <1g; Protein: <1g

Lemony Spinach Pesto

Pesto is a versatile sauce that can be used to top proteins like chicken or fish, roasted vegetables, low-FODMAP toast, roasted potatoes, sweet potatoes, and egg dishes like The Best Hard-Boiled Eggs (page 31) or Creamy Herb-Scrambled Eggs (page 32). Really, most dishes will benefit from being topped with pesto! It's also a nice way to get some more vegetables into your meal in an easily digested form. This recipe works great with either the optional nuts or cheese omitted, but not both.

Makes 1¼ cups

Prep time: 5 minutes

¼ cup garlic oil

¼ cup olive oil

6-ounce bag organic spinach

Grated zest of 1 organic lemon

1 tablespoon freshly squeezed lemon juice

¼ cup chopped pine nuts, walnuts, or almonds (optional)

¼ cup grated Parmesan cheese (optional)

½ teaspoon sea salt

1. In a food processor, combine the garlic oil, olive oil, spinach, lemon zest, lemon juice, nuts (if using), Parmesan cheese (if using), and salt. Process until smooth, stopping to scrape down the sides with a spatula. Taste and add more salt as desired.

2. Serve the pesto immediately or store it in the refrigerator for up to a week.

Ingredient swaps: Instead of spinach, you can use basil in this recipe or another leafy green such as arugula. If you're not using cheese, the mixture will be less salty, so make sure you taste it and add more salt if desired.

Per serving (2 tablespoons): Calories: 100; Total fat: 11g; Saturated fat: 2g; Cholesterol: 0mg; Sodium: 131mg; Carbohydrates: 1g; Sugar: <1g; Fiber: <1g; Protein: 1g

DAIRY-FREE | EGG-FREE | GLUTEN-FREE | NUT-FREE | VEGETARIAN
DIETS: BPD, CSD, GAPS, LFD, SCD, SSFG

Zesty Cilantro Sauce

If you have leftover herbs you need to use up, this sauce takes just minutes to make and adds so much great taste to chicken, beef, pork, fish, and grilled or roasted vegetables. Use it as a dip for low-FODMAP crackers or vegetables, as a sauce for your next Charcuterie & Cheese Board (page 53), or on top of Parchment-Baked Salmon & Potatoes (page 59).

Makes 1 cup

Prep time: 5 minutes

1½ cups packed
    cilantro leaves
⅓ cup red wine vinegar
¼ cup extra-virgin olive oil
¼ cup garlic oil
½ teaspoon sea salt

1. In a food processor, combine the cilantro, vinegar, olive oil, garlic oil, and salt. Blend for about 1 minute or until well mixed, stopping to scrape down the sides as needed. Taste and add more salt as desired.

2. Serve immediately or store in the refrigerator for up to a week.

Ingredient swaps: This sauce is also delicious using parsley leaves instead of cilantro. If you don't tolerate garlic oil, you can leave it out and increase the extra-virgin olive oil to ½ cup.

Per serving (2 tablespoons): Calories: 122; Total fat: 14g; Saturated fat: 2g; Cholesterol: 0mg; Sodium: 149mg; Carbohydrates: <1g; Sugar: 0g; Fiber: <1g; Protein: <1g

Roasted Red Pepper Aioli

This different and delicious aioli is tasty as a dip or in any dish where you would normally use mayonnaise, such as egg salad, tuna salad, or chicken salad. Use this aioli as a spread on a Tomato–Bacon Grilled Cheese Sandwich (page 52) or as a dip for Easy Salmon Cakes (page 57). Raw eggs may contain salmonella and shouldn't be consumed by infants, toddlers, pregnant women, the elderly, or those with compromised immune systems. Purchase raw pasteurized eggs if you fall into one of these categories.

Makes 2 cups

Prep time: 5 minutes

2 large egg yolks

½ teaspoon low-FODMAP mustard (without garlic)

Juice of 1 lemon

1 tablespoon organic tomato paste

½ cup jarred roasted red peppers, drained and chopped

½ teaspoon smoked paprika

½ teaspoon sea salt

½ cup garlic oil

½ cup avocado oil

1. In a food processor, combine the egg yolks, mustard, lemon juice, tomato paste, peppers, paprika, and salt. Process at high speed for 1 minute or until well mixed.

2. With the processor running, slowly pour the garlic oil into the round food pusher. Continue to pour in the garlic oil and then slowly pour in the avocado oil.

3. Scrape the aioli into a bowl and serve it immediately or store it in the refrigerator for up to 3 days.

Speed it up: To make a quicker red pepper aioli, you can use low-FODMAP mayonnaise and mix it in the food processor with the tomato paste, red peppers, and smoked paprika. Taste it and add a little lemon juice and/or salt as desired.

Per serving (2 tablespoons): Calories: 130; Total fat: 14g; Saturated fat: 2g; Cholesterol: 23mg; Sodium: 95mg; Carbohydrates: 1g; Sugar: 1g; Fiber: <1g; Protein: 1g

Tomato Sauce

It's really easy to make your own tomato sauce, and it takes only 30 minutes, so double or triple the recipe and freeze some! This sauce can be served chunky or pureed with a hand blender for a smooth or semi-smooth sauce. Add cooked ground beef or pork sausage if desired and serve over low-FODMAP pasta or vegetable noodles. It also tastes great with the Savory Turkey Meatballs (page 60).

Makes 2½ cups
Prep time: 5 minutes
Cook time: 25 minutes

1 tablespoon olive oil
4 scallions, sliced (green parts only)
1 tablespoon organic tomato paste
1 (26-ounce) container organic chopped tomatoes
¼ cup garlic oil
1 teaspoon fennel seeds
1 tablespoon Italian seasoning (without garlic)
½ teaspoon sea salt

1. In a medium saucepan over medium heat, heat the olive oil for 30 seconds. Add the scallions and sauté for about 2 minutes or until they begin to soften. Add the tomato paste, stir, and cook for 1 minute. Add the chopped tomatoes, garlic oil, fennel seeds, Italian seasoning, and salt. Bring to a simmer and cook for 20 minutes, stirring occasionally.

2. Serve immediately or store in the refrigerator for up to 1 week.

Ingredient swaps: Add capers and kalamata olives to the sauce for a puttanesca-type variation. You can also add finely chopped spinach—it'll disappear into the sauce, and no one will know it's there.

Per serving (½ cup): Calories: 200; Total fat: 16g; Saturated fat: 2g; Cholesterol: 0mg; Sodium: 645mg; Carbohydrates: 15g; Sugar: 8g; Fiber: 3g; Protein: 3g

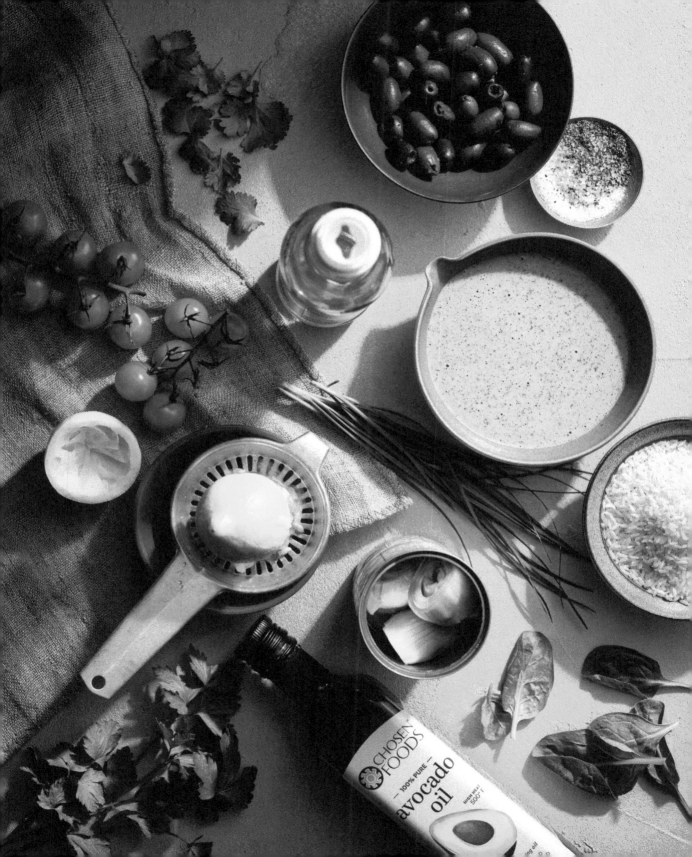

Measurement Conversions

	US STANDARD	US STANDARD (OUNCES)	METRIC (APPROXIMATE)
VOLUME EQUIVALENTS (LIQUID)	2 tablespoons	1 fl. oz.	30 mL
	¼ cup	2 fl. oz.	60 mL
	½ cup	4 fl. oz.	120 mL
	1 cup	8 fl. oz.	240 mL
	1½ cups	12 fl. oz.	355 mL
	2 cups or 1 pint	16 fl. oz.	475 mL
	4 cups or 1 quart	32 fl. oz.	1 L
	1 gallon	128 fl. oz.	4 L
VOLUME EQUIVALENTS (DRY)	⅛ teaspoon	——————	0.5 mL
	¼ teaspoon	——————	1 mL
	½ teaspoon	——————	2 mL
	¾ teaspoon	——————	4 mL
	1 teaspoon	——————	5 mL
	1 tablespoon	——————	15 mL
	¼ cup	——————	59 mL
	⅓ cup	——————	79 mL
	½ cup	——————	118 mL
	⅔ cup	——————	156 mL
	¾ cup	——————	177 mL
	1 cup	——————	235 mL
	2 cups or 1 pint	——————	475 mL
	3 cups	——————	700 mL
	4 cups or 1 quart	——————	1 L
	½ gallon	——————	2 L
	1 gallon	——————	4 L
WEIGHT EQUIVALENTS	½ ounce	——————	15 g
	1 ounce	——————	30 g
	2 ounces	——————	60 g
	4 ounces	——————	115 g
	8 ounces	——————	225 g
	12 ounces	——————	340 g
	16 ounces or 1 pound	——————	455 g

	FAHRENHEIT (F)	CELSIUS (C) (APPROXIMATE)
OVEN TEMPERATURES	250°F	120°C
	300°F	150°C
	325°F	180°C
	375°F	190°C
	400°F	200°C
	425°F	220°C
	450°F	230°C

Resources

Websites

Bristol Stool Scale—BladderAndBowel.org/wp-content/uploads/2017/05/BBC002_Bristol-Stool-Chart-Jan-2016.pdf. A general scale for quality bowel movements.

Clean Fifteen—EWG.org/foodnews/clean-fifteen.php. The Environmental Working Group's guide to 15 fruits and vegetables that contain the lowest concentration of pesticides, which the EWG believes are the safest produce items to buy conventionally.

Dirty Dozen—EWG.org/foodnews/dirty_dozen_list.php#.WI0V8FQ-dTY. The Environmental Working Group's guide to the top 12 fruits and vegetables with the highest concentration of pesticides.

Dr. Allison Siebecker's website—SIBOInfo.com. This site has a wealth of free information about SIBO.

Garlic oil—FODMAPEveryDay.com/know-whats-garlic-oil. An article on why some garlic oils are low-FODMAP and some aren't and which brands are safe to use.

Kristy Regan's site for free SIBO-friendly recipes and information—VitalFoodTherapeutics.com

Monash University FODMAP app—MonashFODMAP.com/i-have-ibs/get-the-app. This app has the most up-to-date and scientifically tested FODMAP list out there.

SIBO Practitioner List from SIBO SOS—Join.SIBOSOS.com/practitioner-list

SIBO SOS Summits, podcasts, online courses, and resources—SIBOSOS.com

The World's Healthiest Foods—WHFoods.com/foodstoc.php. This website offers free scientific-based information on the healthiest foods.

Food Products

24-Hour Yogurt—WMFoods.com/bulgarian-yogurt

Casa de Sante for low-FODMAP stock and broth—casadesante.com /collections/certified-low-fodmap-soup-broth

Collagen hydrolysate—Great Lakes Collagen Hydrolysate or Vital Protein Collagen Peptides, both available on Amazon.com

Great Lakes Gelatin—Available on Amazon.com and in many grocery stores

Low-FODMAP bone broth—GutRxBoneBroth.com

Low-FODMAP prepared foods—FodyFoods.com/collections/all

No-carb, low-alcohol, lower-sulfite, mycotoxin/mold-free wine—DryFarm Wines.com

References

Giaconi, Joann A., Fei Yu, Katie L. Stone, et al. "The Association of Consumption of Fruits/Vegetables with Decreased Risk of Glaucoma among Older African-American Women in the Study of Osteoporotic Fractures." *American Journal of Ophthalmology* 154, no. 4 (October 2012): 635–44.

Huang, Ting-Ting, Jian-Bo Lai, Yan-Li Du, Yi Xu, Lie-Min Ruan, and Shao-Hua Hu. "Current Understanding of Gut Microbiota in Mood Disorders: An Update of Human Studies." *Frontiers in Genetics.* 10, no. 98 (February 2019). doi:10.3389/fgene.2019.00098.

Kerstetter, Jane E., Anne M. Kenny, and Karl L. Insogna. "Dietary Protein and Skeletal Health: A Review of Recent Human Research." *Current Opinion in Lipidology,* 22, no. 1 (2011): 16–20. doi:10.1097/MOL.0b013e3283419441.

Mahendra, Poonam, and Shradha Bisht. "Anti-Anxiety Activity of Coriandrum Sativum Assessed Using Different Experimental Anxiety Models." *Indian Journal of Pharmacology* 43, no. 5 (2011): 574–77. doi:10.4103/0253-7613.84975.

Nehra, Avinash K., et al. "Proton Pump Inhibitors: Review of Emerging Concerns." *Mayo Clinic Proceedings* 93, no. 2 (February 2018): 240–46.

Pimentel, Mark, Evelyn J. Chow, and Henry C. Lin. "Normalization of Lactulose Breath Testing Correlates with Symptom Improvement in Irritable Bowel Syndrome: A Double-Blind, Randomized, Placebo-Controlled Study." *American Journal of Gastroenterology* 98, no. 2 (February 2003): 412–19.

Ingredient Index

Index

Acknowledgments

Thank you to my clients for your bravery. I am honored to be part of your journey.

To Gregg, my husband, best friend, and favorite partner in crime, thank you for making this life such an adventure.

Much gratitude to my family for your ongoing support. Special thanks to my mom for your editing acumen and all your support. I love talking to you about food, writing, nutrition, and life. Thank you to my sister Lisa and brother in-law Jim for being appreciative food testers.

I am so grateful for the community of health providers who I am privileged to work with and learn from. Particular thanks to my colleagues at Hive Mind Medicine, including Dr. Steven Sandberg-Lewis, Kayle Sandberg-Lewis, Dr. Lisa Shaver, Dr. Roz Donovan, Dr. Roxanne Ahmadpour, Dr. Mary Bogle, Dr. Electra Allenton, and Mark Freifeld—I love being part of your community. Thank you to Shivan Sarna for always looking out for me and working so incredibly hard to share SIBO resources with the public. My gratitude to Dr. Allison Siebecker for your wisdom and dedication to the SIBO community. Thank you to my fellow nutritionists Karen David and Marne Minard for sharing your insights and friendship.

I wish I saw my friends more, but I know they are always there for me as I am for them. In particular, thank you to Nichole Alvarado, Nadine Brandon, Brian Durning, Elizabeth Faulkner, Jenn Fieldhack, Jodi Friedman, Kristin Furuichi, Erin Gaffaney, Mary Gelinas, Dani DeMarti (Dani—thank you so much for recommending my books!), Shannon McCaffrey, Andrea Richards, and Robert White.

I'm grateful to everyone at Callisto Media for their patience and assistance through this process.

About the Author

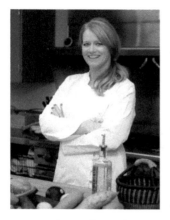

Kristy Regan, MScN, is a holistic nutritionist specializing in therapeutic diets for gastrointestinal disorders as well as other health issues. She practices from a Health at Every Size (HAES) perspective and enjoys supporting her clients in creating a healthy and joyful relationship with food. She studied at National University of Natural Medicine, where she earned her Master of Science in Nutrition degree. Her practice combines nutritional therapy, lifestyle education, and counseling to assist clients in their healing journeys. She appreciates how important it is to connect and address both physical and emotional health. After her own multiyear journey with SIBO, she is able to empathize with her clients and understand their frustrations as well as help them see the light at the end of the tunnel.

Kristy is the author of the books *The SIBO Diet Plan* and *The SIBO Cookbook for the Newly Diagnosed*. Kristy co-organized and spoke at the 2019 NUNM SIBO Symposium. She has been featured on several SIBO SOS online summits.

She is passionate about sharing her expertise in cooking, nutrition, health, and mind–body therapies via podcasts, classes, and speaking engagements. Kristy is available for individual nutrition and wellness appointments online. Visit her website, VitalFoodTherapeutics.com, for free recipes and digestive health information.

CPSIA information can be obtained
at www.ICGtesting.com
Printed in the USA
BVHW091655310821
615706BV00012B/192

9 781647 397364